Evie Graham

This book by Daniel Kennedy and my friend Dr. Francisco Contreras can help all cancer patients learn about the power of the body to heal itself. Standard oncologists ignore this because they do not understand it. They too need to read this book. New studies show that 30 percent of breast cancers seen on mammograms can go away by themselves. We can all make this happen more often if we learn more about the life-saving holistic care provided by the Oasis of Hope Health Group.

–Dr. Garry Gordon
Gordon Research Institute
President and Founder, International College
of Advanced Longevity
Cofounder, American College for Advancement in Medicine

Since 1997 I have supported the work of Dr. Francisco Contreras, Daniel Kennedy, and Oasis of Hope because their approach to cancer is much more comprehensive than mainstream oncology. You will find, as I have, that this book contains many practical tips for beating cancer. I recommend it wholeheartedly.

—Larry MacKay
Founder and President, Cancer Aid and Research Fund

As a pioneer in the alternative therapy movement, Ernesto Contreras Sr., MD, provided *hope* and help to thousands of patients during his long and active practice. In addition, he inspired and mentored many of the physicians who have embraced alternative and integrative therapies in response to the limitations imposed by the conventional, allopathic establishment.

His most devoted and dedicated pupils are his son, Francisco Contreras, MD, and his gr······ Daniel Kennedy, MC. Through their efforts, they transform······ into a world-class medical facility that s······ g alternative therapies with the best conv······

Dr. Contreras and Dani······ coauthored a number of books, written to assist both pati······ cians. *Beating Cancer* is the latest contribution. This book is not a stand-alone self-treatment guide but a self-help resource for patients in their journey toward healing. Just as Dr. Contreras Sr. was a pioneer in bringing integration—body, mind, and spirit—to cancer therapy, his son and grandson extend his legacy to new generations of cancer patients.

Practical, thorough, and based on forty-eight years of treating tens of thousands of cancer patients from around the world, *Beating Cancer* has much to offer cancer patients, their families, and the physicians who treat them.

—Frank Cousineau
President, Cancer Control Society and
International Association of Cancer Victors and Friends

Conventional cancer treatment does not give much hope. Dr. Contreras's integrative approach to cancer does. If you or a loved one has cancer, read this book. You will be introduced to a whole different way to fight cancer, a way that has helped tens of thousands of people over the last five decades.

—William Lee Cowden, MD, MD(H)
Chairman, The Scientific Advisory Board
Academy of Comprehensive Integrative Medicine

Beating
Cancer

20 Natural, Spiritual, & Medical Remedies

that can slow—and even reverse—cancer's progression

FRANCISCO **CONTRERAS**, MD

Expert on cancer therapies and chairman
of the Oasis of Hope Health Group

DANIEL **KENNEDY**, MC

Spiritual and emotional life director and
CEO of the Oasis of Hope Health Group

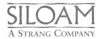

SILOAM
A STRANG COMPANY

Most STRANG COMMUNICATIONS BOOK GROUP products are available at special quantity discounts for bulk purchase for sales promotions, premiums, fund-raising, and educational needs. For details, write Strang Communications Book Group, 600 Rinehart Road, Lake Mary, Florida 32746, or telephone (407) 333-0600.

BEATING CANCER by Francisco Contreras, MD, and Daniel E. Kennedy
Published by Siloam, A Strang Company
600 Rinehart Road, Lake Mary, Florida 32746
www.strangbookgroup.com

Scripture quotations marked KJV are from the King James Version of the Bible.

Scripture quotations marked NAS are from the New American Standard Bible. Copyright © 1960, 1962, 1963, 1968, 1971, 1972, 1973, 1975, 1977, 1995 by the Lockman Foundation. Used by permission. (www.Lockman.org)

Scripture quotations marked NIV are from the Holy Bible, New International Version. Copyright © 1973, 1978, 1984, International Bible Society. Used by permission.

Design Director: Bill Johnson
Cover design by Judith Wright

Visit the authors' website at www.oasisofhope.com.

Library of Congress Cataloging-in-Publication Data:
Contreras, Francisco.
    Beating cancer / Francisco Contreras And Daniel E. Kennedy.
        p. cm.
    Previously published: Fighting cancer 20 different ways, c2005.
    Includes bibliographical references.
    ISBN 978-1-61638-156-1
    1. Cancer--Popular works. 2. Cancer--Prevention. I. Kennedy, Daniel E.
II. Contreras, Francisco. Fighting cancer 20 different ways. III. Title.
    RC263.C6483 2010
    616.99'4--dc22
                                            2010037858

E-book ISBN: 1-978-61638-411-1

The first edition of this book was published as *Fighting Cancer 20 Different Ways* (Siloam, 2005). Portions of this book were previously published in *The Hope of Living Cancer Free* (Siloam, 1999), ISBN 0-88419-655-0, and *The Coming Cancer Cure* (Siloam, 2002), ISBN 0-88419-846-4.

11 12 13 14 15 — 9 8 7 6 5 4 3 2 1
Printed in the United States of America

DEDICATION

T o those who are on the cancer journey: May courage, faith, hope, and love be your companions. May you soar like eagles and find refuge in the shadow of His wings. The adventures along the path are more rewarding than reaching the destination.

ACKNOWLEDGMENTS

E WISH TO ACKNOWLEDGE AND THANK A NUMBER OF people who have been instrumental in the development of the concepts shared in this book and the publishing of this book. We thank the thousands of patients and their families who have shared their lives, experience, and wisdom with us. You have been our most important teachers. We thank Stephen Strang for partnering with us in our mission to improve the quality of the physical, spiritual, and emotional lives of people around the world. Thanks to the team at Strang Communications and the wonderful editors, designers, marketers, and public relation teams that are making it possible for this book to reach the hands of those who will benefit from it. Thanks to the incredible research and administrative teams at the Oasis of Hope, including Dr. Jorge Barroso-Aranda, Mark McCarty, Leticia Wong, Michael Wood, Luisa Ruiz, Mary Bernal, and Tom Klaber. In all things, to God be the glory!

In addition, Daniel Kennedy writes the following: Thank you, Veronica, Estela, and Daniella, for your love, commitment, inspiration, and sacrifice. Dad, my best friend, you have taught me many things, including what victory over cancer looks like.

CONTENTS

NOTE TO THE READER

THIS BOOK WAS WRITTEN BY TWO MEN, FRANCISCO CONTRERAS, MD, and Daniel E. Kennedy, who oversee the Oasis of Hope cancer treatment centers in southern California and Mexico. Dr. Contreras is a surgical oncologist and has been the president and chairman of the Oasis of Hope Health Group since 1983. He brings more than twenty-seven years of practical experience and clinical research to the fight against cancer.

Daniel Kennedy is the chief executive officer of the Oasis of Hope Health Group and has been counseling cancer patients since 1993, emphasizing the emotional, psychological, and spiritual strategies for fighting cancer. He holds degrees in counseling, ministry, economics, and business. Daniel Kennedy is also the nephew of Dr. Contreras.

Together they bring you a full arsenal of ways to come against cancer. Although both authors worked closely together on this entire book, you'll find that some chapters are written in Dr. Contreras's voice and some are written in Daniel Kennedy's voice, since each author brings a unique perspective and specialized focus. For your convenience, the publisher has indicated who is speaking in parentheses near the beginning of each chapter.

About the Details

No one person can know all the words specific to all aspects of modern medical science, no matter how well read he or she might be. As a result, one of the most difficult decisions in preparing this resource involved the use of medical and scientific terms that might not be familiar to many readers, even those of a scientific bent.

Electing to walk a middle path as much as possible is the course chosen for this book. So, on the one hand you will sometimes read unfamiliar words in the text in places where they simply cannot be avoided. When you encounter these, we urge you not to give up. The underlying concept is always more important than the specific vocabulary.

In other places the more technical discussions were moved to the Notes at the end of this book, keyed to numbers within the text itself. So if you want more information and you don't mind academic language, we have it there for you.

INTRODUCTION

O<small>N</small> S<small>EPTEMBER</small> 12, 1962, P<small>RESIDENT</small> J<small>OHN</small> F. K<small>ENNEDY</small> confidently declared, "We choose to go to the moon." He believed that America had the brainpower and the will to achieve anything we set our sites on if we would fund the project adequately. He stated that it was critical for the United States of America to lead the world in space exploration and be the first to send a man to the moon. Less than five years later, in the summer of 1969, the historic words came forth from Neil Armstrong: "It's one small step for man; one giant leap for mankind." At that moment, as the world witnessed humans walking on the moon, there was a belief that anything could be achieved. President Kennedy's leadership and policies made the conquering of outer space possible.

In 1971, President Richard Nixon set out to topple one of the most perplexing and devastating mutations of inner space—cancer. He declared the war on cancer and signed the National Cancer Act, which funded a new research division of the National Institutes of Health (NIH) called the National Cancer Institute (NCI).[1] President Nixon believed that America had the brainpower and will to lead the world and be the first to find the cure to cancer. That would be a giant leap for mankind, much greater than a lunar trip.

As we reach the forty-year mark since the war on cancer was declared and after hundreds of billions of dollars have been spent on research, treatment, and education, are we any closer to beating cancer? Here are the cold numbers that we face today. According to the NCI, nearly 1.5 million people will be diagnosed with cancer in the United States this year. Close to six hundred thousand Americans will die from it just this year alone. If you live in the United States, the probability that you will be diagnosed with cancer sometime during your life is 1 in 3.[2] The cure to cancer has not been found.

The best and brightest in the medical community need to embrace a different approach. This was never clearer to me than when I was a medical student. My late father, Dr. Ernesto Contreras Sr., was accepted as a keynote speaker at a world congress on cancer, subject to a peer review by oncologists at the famed Memorial Sloan-Kettering Cancer Center in New York.

At the start of our meeting, my father put up a diagnostic chest X-ray alongside a post-treatment X-ray of one of our patients, with both X-rays showing a tumor. One of the oncologists, apparently perturbed, stood up and said, "That's not a successful case."

He left the room and returned with X-rays of one of his own patients. The diagnostic X-ray showed a tumor, and the post-treatment X-ray did not. My father congratulated the doctor and asked how the patient was doing. The oncologist said, "The patient died, but the treatment was successful."

My father pointed out that even though cancer was still present in the X-rays he presented, the X-rays were taken ten years apart, and the patient continued to live and work with the cancer completely under control.

The Memorial Sloan-Kettering oncologist, like many other doctors, treated the tumor, not the patient. Destruction of the tumor was the measure of success with little or no regard to whether or not the patient survived. Conventional medicine remains infatuated with eradicating the tumor and winning the war on cancer, when instead it should be looking at the total patient and fighting the battle one patient at a time.

Though there is not much promise emanating from the hallowed halls of research, there are specific steps you can take to push closer to your personal goal of beating cancer. The keys to victory are hidden within three errors in the cancer research and treatment models:

1. Researchers have tried to identify *the cure* (singular) to cancer. They test isolated drugs and measure tumor reduction. This is not in line with reality because cancer is systemic, and no single drug will ever address the multiple needs of each system in the body. Researchers must shift and consider integrative treatment modalities.

2. Doctors are reactive and treat symptoms. Oncologists can no longer focus on the tumor; they must focus on the whole patient: body, soul, and spirit. They must get to the roots of cancer instead of dealing with its symptoms. A tumor is the consequence of an unhealthy person; the tumor is not the disease to be dealt with.

3. Patients are passive in their treatment. A person should not lie back and let the doctors and nurses try to cure them. Instead, the patient must be active and do everything possible to help the doctor help him or her beat cancer.

Making these three changes is the kind of health-care reform that will really add years of abundant living to people's life. Our researchers have developed treatment modalities that support the whole patient and tear down cancer from every possible angle. Our doctors are proactive and don't depend solely on the standard drug therapy. As one of our oncologists stated, "If you want textbook results, use textbook therapies." Well, we have looked at the statistics, and we are not willing to ask our patients to settle for textbook results. We go way above and beyond the standard of care to the level that the patient needs. The standard of care is a starting place, not a goal to be achieved. We work with our patients and recognize that they are the captains of their treatment teams, and we teach them how to change their lives and close the door on cancer.

Prevention vs. Treatment

You may wonder why we discuss prevention and treatment of cancer in the same book. Hippocrates stated that "your food shall be your medicine and that your medicine shall be your food." The unavoidable implication is that whatever is good to *prevent* is also good to *treat*. This 2,300-year-old principle is still true today. Prevention principles, integrated to a specific therapy, are quite applicable and helpful to even advanced cancer patients.

We also address both prevention and treatment because we know that patients who've been treated for cancer—and their loved ones—are the best advocates for prevention. At Oasis of Hope, we spend hours every day educating patients on how to beat cancer, and ever since Dr. Ernesto Contreras Sr. founded the hospital in 1963, we have invited a companion to participate in the educational program at no additional charge. Since most companions are family members, which means they are related to someone who has cancer, they really need to take steps to prevent cancer, not necessarily because they have similar genes but because they likely have the same lifestyle. We believe that everyone who has cancer and reads this book should get a copy into the hands of loved ones to help them beat cancer before it starts.

Different Treatments for Different Cancers

Even though there are many types of cancers with varying degrees of aggression, there is no question that there also are some common denominators to all of them. These commonalities are the heart of this book; these principles will give you resources to beat all odds.

We wanted this book to be relevant to you regardless of the type of cancer you need to beat. So we are presenting the principles and steps you could take no matter what the diagnosis is. The purpose of this book is to help you help your doctor so that together, you can beat cancer. It is not intended to be a guide to self-medicating. We believe that if you are doing everything that we share, and you work closely with an integrative oncologist who can provide a comprehensive integrated program, you will increase your probability of beating cancer, and you may diminish negative side effects and fill your life with more meaningful experiences.

This book will provide you with twenty specific things you can do to beat cancer. But nothing in the battle against cancer happens in isolation. Likewise, none of the twenty ways to beat cancer should be allowed to stand entirely alone. Taken together, these tactics for battling or preventing cancer form up like a battle line of well-trained soldiers united in one purpose: to give you a fighting chance against cancer. This multifocal approach to beating cancer is based on forty-eight years of clinical experience treating more than one hundred thousand patients who have come to Oasis of Hope from fifty-five nations.

How Is This Book Put Together?

The whole point in writing this book is to bring together in one place an effective battle plan that you can put into action in your own fight against cancer. But before you can pick out your weapons, you have to know your enemy. You also need to understand how the battle has been fought so far. That's what section one, "Preparing for Battle," is all about. There you'll find the explanation of how cancer starts, how it spreads, and how it can sometimes be stalled or defeated by medical or surgical responses.

The heart of this book, section two, "Twenty Ways to Beat Cancer," then presents a series of practical ways to help you begin fighting cancer right now. Accompanied by plenty of supporting evidence, these twenty cancer-beating strategies are discussed for the remaining chapters of the book.

As you progress through the twenty cancer beaters, you'll find three main categories. Cancer-beating steps one through ten include the *physical* things you can do yourself through diet and lifestyle choices that will directly affect the way your body can resist cancer.

Cancer-beating steps eleven through sixteen highlight the ways you can further improve your resistance by mounting a powerful, two-pronged offensive centered in your *emotions* and your *will*.

Cancer-beating steps seventeen through twenty look at what are truly the most powerful weapons of all, the *spiritual* resources you can deploy in harmony with all the above. These spiritual resources are also those you can rest in, rely on, and refresh yourself with for as long as you draw breath and then through eternity as well.

Because you've picked up this book, it's likely that cancer has invaded your life. Whether its effects are direct (you personally) or indirect (someone you love), you want to fight it, you want to take an active stance, and you want to *beat* it. The ultimate goal of *Beating Cancer* is to help you do all you can do to send this invader back where it came from.

Oasis of Hope is caring for the whole person: body, soul, and spirit; sharing the healing power of faith, hope, and love; and advancing science and medicine to put an end to cancer, one person at a time. As a part of our mission, we are reaching out to you with this book. Our goal is to empower you to work together more effectively with your physicians and health professionals so that you can start beating cancer.

Let's get started.

SECTION I
PREPARING FOR BATTLE

My people are destroyed from lack of knowledge.
—HOSEA 4:6, NIV

BEFORE YOU CAN UNDERSTAND THE TWENTY-PLUS WAYS OF fighting cancer, you need to understand a little about how cancer works and what is typically done to combat it. Once you have that under your belt, you'll be able to see how the twenty cancer-beating strategies in this book fit in.

It's amazing to think about all the wrong information that's out there. Correcting these misunderstandings is a frequent part of consultation with patients at the Oasis of Hope treatment centers. There will be some myth-busting in the book too.

Here are some of the common medical myths targeted by the writing of this book:

- Myth #1: Cancer is a death sentence.

- Myth #2: The cure for cancer will be found soon if we raise enough research money.

- Myth #3: Radical mastectomies are more effective than lumpectomies.

- Myth #4: Nutrition and lifestyle have nothing to do with preventing or reversing cancer.

- Myth #5: Emotional and spiritual therapies boost morale but do not help the body heal.

- Myth #6: Tumor eradication is the only acceptable outcome of cancer treatment.

- Myth #7: Chemotherapy is effective in most cancers.

- Myth #8: Cancer is a matter of chance—you either get it or you don't.

- Myth #9: All alternative medicine is quackery.

- Myth #10: Mammograms prevent breast cancer.

- Myth #11: If you have the cancer gene, you will get cancer.

- Myth #12: If you have cancer, you cannot do anything to improve your chances to survive.

Given how many people believe this "misinformation," perhaps it's no wonder that millions perish from cancer every year. Fear alone has a powerful negative influence. But it doesn't have to affect you that way. Truly, *where there is life there is hope!*

Oasis of Hope[1] is attacking cancer in every possible way and proving, over and over again, in the lives of patients who come from all over the world, that a multidimensional approach to cancer treatment and prevention can work wonders.

Since writing this book as *Fighting Cancer 20 Different Ways* in 2005, a few things have changed. The principles of this book are solid; nevertheless, new technologies and research are uncovering elements with new information that have helped us fine-tune our message and therapies. Therefore we felt the need to share this deeper understanding through an update of our book.

It has been exciting to see how much information is coming out of the research forums on how to overcome the weaknesses of chemotherapy, surgery, and radiation through natural therapies. Even as recently as the last few years, many studies are being conducted using elements such as green tea and vitamin C. As little as ten years ago, Oasis of Hope and the Contreras doctors were often criticized for our use of natural therapies. Now we are being validated as the scientific community is proving the value. Due to the emergence of such studies in the medical literature, we have been able to evolve as a treatment center and fine-tune our protocols.

In the same way, the message of *Beating Cancer* has been updated to reflect the latest treatments and therapies, yet one thing remains the same: the goal is to put you in the driver's seat. But that can't happen unless you are willing to consider the following truths:

1. First, licensed medical doctors should always be an extremely important part of your healing equation. You need them on your team. No one should ever try to face cancer without a great deal of professional help. You should have at least one oncologist on your team as well as an integrative medicine specialist. A nutritionist, along with emotional and spiritual counselors, are extremely important as well.

2. Second, if you are faced with cancer, the other important player on your personal healing team is you. Indeed, you are by far the most important person in the healing process. As this book will show you, you have more power than you might think.

3. Third, regardless of how much knowledge, skill, and wisdom you and your doctors bring to your situation, the same God who created all of us remains the sovereign author of life and the ultimate healer. Sometimes He even helps people who don't believe He exists, but having seen up close and personal what He can do, it is impossible to share that lack of belief! God has declared that no man

shall be without excuse, which applies with awesome
power to those who watch Him at work every day.

The following chapters will demonstrate that cancer is a vicious disease. But it can be fought. It must be beaten!

And God has given us many weapons.

Chapter 1

O PARADIGM, O PARADIGM!

I(Francisco Contreras) must have been daydreaming, but the vision in my mind certainly seemed real. I saw a beautiful ten-year-old girl staring at me over the nameplate on my desk: *Dr. Francisco Contreras, Surgical Oncologist.*

"My name is Sarah. Who are you?"

"I am Dr. Contreras," I replied. "And who are you?"

At that point I quickly reviewed Sarah's case notes and began to interview her and her parents. Ever since Sarah first noticed a big lump on her arm a year or so before, she had spent more time in medical institutions than at school or at home. She had already endured one surgery, after which she had hoped that everything would again be all right.

Yet her parents still acted strangely when she was around. They weren't as strict as they'd once been, and they spent many hours behind closed doors crying. Sarah began to wonder if the big term the doctor had used to explain her problem had upset her parents. It took her weeks to learn how to pronounce and spell it: non-Hodgkin's lymphoma.

Whatever it was, Sarah knew it wasn't good. Her parents told her, "The doctors are offering you chemotherapy, but they said it wouldn't help you much. What do you want to do?"

"I know I am in God's hands, and I have peace," Sarah replied.

Her parents decided to look for a different approach. That is when Sarah became our patient at Oasis of Hope.

"Dr. Contreras…Dr. Contreras…Dr. Contreras…"

Suddenly, I snapped out of my daydream in response to the voice of an angelic vision of beauty standing before me dressed in a wedding gown. It was Sarah! "Can it be true that twelve years have passed since God delivered Sarah from cancer?" I asked myself. My wife and I then took our seats to witness one of the most inspiring weddings we have ever attended.

All of Sarah's family and friends were there. We were sitting in the next-to-the-last pew, where I suddenly found myself crying so uncontrollably I began to worry that I'd use up all the moisture in my body. The joy I felt was overwhelming.

Soon Sarah stood at the altar with the young man of her dreams, who immediately became the envy of every bachelor who had ever met Sarah. I only wished that I had a son old enough to marry this lovely, talented, sweet young woman, thus bringing her forever into my own family!

Sarah credits God, her parents, and my father, Dr. Ernesto Contreras Sr., for her victory over cancer. She is right to do so, but I would add to that list her own determination, starting when she was just a little girl. She now is a college graduate and serves the Lord with her husband, who is the pastor of their youth group. They also have a precious little boy.

How was she able to overcome the insurmountable? Four words come to mind: openness, flexibility, adaptability, and commitment. Sarah and her parents looked beyond the tunnel-vision, chemotherapeutic attack on cancer that had already failed. They opened themselves up to other options. They were flexible and willing to try new treatments. They were able to adapt to different circumstances.

Above all else, they were totally committed to seeing Sarah well again. And perhaps all of that, taken together, explains why they were able to embrace an eclectic, multifaceted approach that depended on them every bit as much as it did on the doctors.

It All Begins With Philosophy

Sometimes chemotherapy and radiation work, and sometimes they don't. If you and your doctor subscribe to the philosophy that you will have no hope if the medicine doesn't work, then you won't have any such hope. Your philosophy will either limit your possibilities or open them up.

My point is that everything begins and ends with philosophy—the paradigm by which we frame every aspect of our existence, the filter that helps us to decide how and what we think. If you doubt, simply consider the entire academic world. It doesn't matter what field a person might choose; the highest degree is a Doctor of Philosophy (abbreviated as PhD). You can get a PhD in immunology, anthropology, mathematics, literature, and many other disciplines as well.

Perhaps as a natural consequence, the philosophy of medicine, as birthed in the early twentieth century, has evolved into the treatment paradigm of the twenty-first century. Think about that for a moment! The twentieth century was an era of scientific breakthrough and technological advance, yet we began it without electricity, television, airplanes, and computers.

The scientific and technological revolutions of the twentieth century had a profound impact on the medical field as well. Scientists developed an arsenal of pharmaceuticals designed to address just about every pathogen. Meanwhile, even as I write these words, new technologies such as lasers, 3-D imaging devices, proton therapy, robotic surgery, DNA laboratory exams, cyberknives, and fiber-optic cameras are assisting physicians in the field. The results of all these advances have been impressive.

For example, acute medicine is now at the top of its game. Doctors can save life and limb in ways never before thought possible. If Humpty Dumpty had been brought to a modern trauma center, he would have gone back together in no time at all.

In addition, once-complex medical procedures such as angioplasty and open-heart surgery have now become routine. People don't fret anywhere near as much as they used to when they go under the knife. Technology has transformed the operating room into a much more controlled environment than ever before.

Overall, we owe the scientific method for most of the important advances in medicine. Science has awed all of us at one time or another, and it continues to do so on a regular basis. The development of scientific methodology has evolved to such an extent that not even the sky is the limit anymore. In fact, every month I put some money in my piggybank because I want to go on the first commercial trip to outer space!

Inner space has been no match for scientific methodology either. It took less than two decades for scientists to unravel the trillions of letters of the human genome, the code of life.

Again, most projects like that have conquered outer and inner space because of vision, intelligence, planning, and perseverance, combined with adequate funding and strict adherence to scientific methods. Thus many tasks once thought impossible have now been made almost routine.

But somewhere in the shadow of all these scientific victories, cancer still lurks as the unconquered enemy. Hundreds of years after it was first identified, cancer in most (or all) of its forms still manages to evade, elude, and confound the best efforts of the best scientists.

The Old Way Just Doesn't Work!

When faced with monumental challenges, scientists of all disciplines must first learn all they can about what they want to conquer—the moon, bacteria, or cancer. Experts of all disciplines generally evaluate each challenge through a process called SWOT (strengths, weaknesses, opportunities, and threats). They analyze everything on both sides of the equation, including their own SWOTs, before they can hope to map out a strategic action plan.

As in conventional warfare, scientific theory says that the side with more strengths and opportunities should overcome the side with the most weaknesses and the least chance to evade and avoid threats. Yet until now, cancer has defied everything that science has thrown at it. It has dodged or defeated every hopeful advance. After four decades of tireless efforts by countless scientists around the world spending hundreds of billions of research dollars, the conquest of cancer still seems out of reach.

Is all this true because the scientific method is not as effective as we once thought? Or is it because cancer's strengths are insurmountable?

My answer to both questions is an emphatic no! I am convinced that tackling cancer from a different perspective will generate positive results. Current treatment and research paradigms have literally become the problem, as embodied within two fundamental aspects of that framework: (1) the methods and (2) the goals of modern research.

Many of the treatments being explored today do not have as their goal a complete cure for cancer. Instead, the goal is a drug treatment to hinder and slow the progress of this dreaded disease. While drug treatments can lessen the impact of cancer, making it a chronic disease that does not end in death, it is important to remember that there are no "magic bullets."

Put another way, I feel the goal of pharmaceutical companies and the U.S. Food and Drug Administration (FDA) is to isolate the single agent that could bring about "the cure." But cancer has many different causes. Therefore there is no one substance that will cure it in all instances and in all people. We must use great caution when applying new drug therapies and never forget the need for personally tailored medical treatment.

Will Health-Care Reform Be the Answer?

I'm sure that with the health-care reform currently being enacted, more Americans will have access to medical management, but inevitably it also means that the care will be diluted. For instance, in England many drugs available in the United States are off limits, and waiting time for doctor's appointments, scheduled scans and surgeries, etc. are quite long. Now more than ever we should take responsibility for our health and do all we can to prevent loss of our health through preventive measures in order to depend as little as possible on government health-care systems.

Health-care reform is a topic that I watch carefully. I am always on alert of how government regulation will limit or improve my ability to help patients beat cancer. I believe that many more people could be cured of cancer just through health-care reform. I am tempted to get excited when I hear politicians begin to take on the challenge of reforming how health care is delivered. But the sad reality is that it really isn't about health-care reform. It is really about payer reform, that is to say, *who* is going to pay, *how* it will be paid, and *what* will be paid for.

When the focus is about the payment of health care, the care made available to patients usually is brought down to the least common denominator. I have seen this firsthand in Mexico where medicine is socialized, which means the government runs the hospitals and everybody has equal access to health care. But the reality is that while everybody has equal access, not everybody has access to equal levels of treatment. To get the latest cancer treatments, which are always the most expensive drugs, only people who can go outside of the system and pay cash will have the chance to get those treatments. The government-run hospitals have limited resources that have to be spread out to cover everybody. This limits patients' access to the best treatments.

Imagine that you have prepared soup for ten people, but one hundred arrived, and you have no more ingredients. You may have to add a lot of water. Now the nutritional value each of the one hundred receives is far less than what the original ten would have received. Watered-down health care is what will be delivered if the focus on health-care reform continues to be about who will pay what.

The health-care reform that we need should be focused on health. We need to start changing our research funding policies. Today, the National Cancer Institute (NCI), a branch of the National Institutes of Health (NIH), dedicates less than 2 percent of its budget to researching how to prevent cancer. This is tragic because every year, the incidence of cancer increases. The amount of money spent on treatment continues to balloon because more and more people are getting sick. The true cure to cancer is to never get it at all. If more research dollars were spent on prevention, and preventative measures were found and implemented, there would be hope for fewer people ever getting cancer. The money spent on treatment would then decline and the vicious cycle could be broken.

The other shift in research that is needed is for fewer studies to be done on drug therapies and more studies to be done on natural therapies. I am enthusiastic because there are more studies underway in the arena of natural therapies at major institutions than ever before.

The biggest way to improve how patients are treated would be to do away with malpractice insurance. The best high-wire artists have always been the ones who have walked that narrow path without a safety net. If a doctor is treating you without the malpractice safety net, he or she will spend more time with you to make sure you receive the highest quality of care as well as the friendliest care. But listen, I am a doctor, so I am not coming against doctors with this suggestion. I am really against the system that rewards money for improper or negligent health care. It should not be about the money. It should be about the quality of health care. If a patient or the family member feels that the care was negligent or even criminal, the claim should be made to the medical boards and it should be about the physician's license, not about cash awards. If the medical board would find the doctor guilty of malpractice, his or her license could be revoked or suspended until the physician received further training and correction. This would bring the focus back to health care, not money.

Even as I am writing this, I am just two days away from a visit from Patch Adams to the Oasis of Hope. In his dream hospital, no doctor would ever be allowed to carry malpractice insurance. He believes that doctors must become real friends with a patient and that a patient would never sue the doctor if they knew that the doctor really cared for them. Patch and I will have a conversation on camera on the healing power of the doctor-patient relationship, and by the time this book gets into your hand, you will be able to see the video online at www.oasisofhope.com. Please visit the website and watch the video. I am sure that it will be quite interesting.

Where Are We Going, and How Will We Get There?

In the spring of 2004, *Fortune* magazine featured a riveting cover of solid black with a big red headline: "Why We Are Losing the War Against Cancer." The subtitle added, "And How We Can Win It." My immediate reaction was to wonder why they had taken such a negative approach. I was well aware of how badly we need to get the upper hand, but even I was shocked to read their inside information on cancer research.

The author explained that more than $14 billion in private and government funds are spent in America every year on searching for the cure, but little progress has been made. Each research project is managed independently, and the various research centers do not share information with one another.

Remember the story of the six blind men trying to describe an elephant? Each man touches a different part of the elephant, such as the leg, tail, and tusk. They then describe the elephant based on the one part that they felt and discover they completely disagree with each other. The story illustrates the misconceptions that can come about when a person's perspective is limited to one small piece of a bigger picture. Clearly, no one in cancer research is working with the big picture. And yet, according to *Fortune*, we could win the war against cancer if the National Institutes of Health would obligate researchers to share information and coordinate their efforts.

Sadly, I agree that more information sharing would be beneficial, but I doubt that one single remedy would be enough. The more basic problem is that researchers are starting from the wrong place, and they're aiming for a destination that probably doesn't exist. Let me repeat what I hope I have already made plain: I don't think the cure to cancer exists in the form of one substance, technique, or apparatus. I do believe that cancer can be defeated, but only through a multifaceted, eclectic approach.

Let me rephrase this in simpler terms. The search for a magic bullet is a waste of time and resources. It is tantamount to chasing rainbows, hoping to find that elusive pot of gold at the end.

Such an approach reminds me of the always-broke investors who aim only for the "big score," in contrast to the professionals who take a little bit of profit from every little trade and wind up rich.

Likewise, science has uncovered many, many things that can diminish the power of cancer, but the goal of many in the research community remains that one huge score.

Our goal is to share with you the many "small" things you can do to minimize cancer's advantages. This means you must consider your doctor a member of your treatment team, not your boss. You must take responsibility for your own health and make informed decisions. Do not accept the status quo!

Approach cancer from every viable angle you can identify. In so doing you will develop a powerful personal philosophy, and you will put policies in place that will serve you well in your mission to undermine cancer.

That is precisely what Sarah and her parents did, and it worked. She has now been free of cancer for more than twenty years.

Chapter 2

GENETIC INSTABILITY

IF YOU COULD LIVE ANYWHERE IN THE WORLD, WHERE WOULD IT be? For me (Francisco Contreras), Paris sits at the top of the list. Nothing compares with walking down the Champs-Elysées in the evening, toward the beautifully lit l'Arc de Triomphe with the Eiffel Tower in the distance. I love sitting in a quaint café on the avenue with my wife, waiting to see if the waiter lives up to the fabulous reputation of Parisian servers. And no visit to Paris would be complete without spending a morning at the Louvre Museum, home of the *Venus de Milo* and da Vinci's *Mona Lisa*, perhaps followed by a visit to the Notre Dame Cathedral and a late lunch on the water, cruising down the Seine River.

Paris is one of the most coveted cities in the world. Throughout history, all the great conquerors of the Western world have wished to add France to their empires. And they all knew that when Paris fell, the whole of France would soon surrender too.

Things would be much the same in the battle against cancer if we could conquer genetic instability. If we could stabilize genes, everything else would become moot, because cancer isn't cancer without cell mutation. And cell mutation occurs because of genetic instability.

But right here is also what makes it such a huge challenge. Thousands of factors can cause genes to become unstable and allow cells to mutate. So let's begin with that.

What Are We Dealing With Here?

The United States government created the National Cancer Institute (NCI) in 1937, with sponsorship from every senator in Congress. This unusual agreement among lawmakers reflected the nation's growing concern about cancer. The NCI was authorized to award grants to non-federal scientists for research on cancer and to fund fellowships for researchers.[1]

Unfortunately, the NCI's initial efforts were not sufficient, so thirty-four years later, in 1971, President Richard Nixon signed the National Cancer Act into law. This bold legislation mobilized even more of the country's resources to fight cancer and infused enough dollars and authority into the NCI to make, in Nixon's words, "the conquest of cancer a national crusade."[2]

Nearly forty years later, exasperated critics and millions of cancer patients do not understand why we can put a man on the moon in only eleven years, yet through seven decades of research during which the USA—and many other countries—have provided unrestricted funds for an army of the most brilliant minds to wage war against cancer, a cure has not been found.

Supporters say that this long crusade has been fruitful. Thanks to the indefatigable efforts of researchers, we have learned a lot about cancer. And yet, while it's possible that the knowledge so far acquired might someday form the foundation for the long-awaited cure, we still cannot wipe it out.

The basic argument is that cancer is a challenge like no other because of its unpredictability, its ability to change and adapt, its resilience (i.e., its "comeback" ability), and its destructiveness. All these traits make up cancer's strengths, which are made even stronger by the chaos in its developmental core. While normal tissue growth and development are based on structured, predictable, and precise transfers of information from mother to daughter cells through the DNA (i.e., the blueprint), cancer's DNA is riddled with mutations, causing devastating errors in information transmission. Scientists call the resulting chaos genetic instability.[3]

The Telephone Game

Have you ever played the telephone game? A group of people sit in a line, and the first person whispers a sentence into the next person's ear. That person is supposed to whisper the same sentence to the next person, and the next person whispers it to the next, and so on until the end of the line is reached.

Let's say that the sentence, "My dog has fleas," was the original. The game sounds easy enough, but inevitably the sentence morphs into something like, "My cat can sneeze." That's funny, but faulty replication is no laughing matter when your life depends on accurate, old-cell-to-new-cell duplication.

To illustrate the concept even more graphically, let's take the following message, which could save the world if it could be shared (i.e., replicated) effectively.

Original message:
Love heals; hate kills; forgive and forget.

Perfect replication of the message:
Love heals; hate kills; forgive and forget.

Mismatch or translocation:
Love kills; hate heals; forgive and forget.

Large deletions:
Love kills, and forget.

An Imperfect Analogy

See how a few simple replication errors, however small, can change a message of hope into a call for World War III? Now apply the concept to cancerous cells. A malignant tissue is made up of many different types of mutated cells. Moreover, the mutations never stop and are absolutely unpredictable!

How do these mutations get started? Well, among the trillions of normal cells in our bodies, unimaginable numbers of cell divisions for regeneration are constantly taking place. Information replication errors (mutations) are not uncommon, but our system is generally capable of correcting them. We all have special genes called mismatch repair genes. These genes are part of the intricate molecular machinery, a sort of "genetic Liquid Paper" that automatically fixes the cellular DNA when, for some reason, cell replication doesn't quite work correctly.

But when mismatch repair genes do not do their job, the result is often cancer.

It has been a long and tedious undertaking to try to understand how genetic instability arises in the common human cancers. For many years the main goal of most cancer research has been to identify the specific genes responsible for it. If we could do that, according to the prevailing research paradigm, we'd have a chance to find a cure. After all, if you'll pardon the simplistic comparison, you can't design either a defense or an offense against your opponent until you know how he plays the game.

On the other hand, your opponent can't win if you always score more points. This is a crude and imperfect analogy, but perhaps it can partially explain why I think we should look first at how we might be able to "outscore" cancer by restoring stability within and among the cells that are running amok.

Restoring Stability

As I've already indicated, based on the sheer volume of information sharing going on within our bodies, a certain percentage of cell-to-cell transcription errors simply have to be expected. Remember, the body has its own "genetic Liquid Paper" to correct such errors, which we wouldn't need if errors were not part of the normal equation.

How does this "genetic Liquid Paper" work? Well, a mismatch repair gene is a protein complex found in healthy human cells. Its first protein attaches to mismatched information (called nucleotides). Then, its second protein takes charge and orchestrates the correction of these errors.[4]

Again, this example is vastly oversimplified, but it's a little like the forestry teams who work through a stand of timber thinning out diseased trees so the healthy ones can survive. The advance man marks the trees that have to come out, while the men with the chain saws come behind and make the actual correction.

Another way of looking at genetic instability, then, is to understand that insufficient levels of the two essential proteins are an important part of the problem. If you don't have enough "genetic Liquid Paper" on hand, errors accumulate and cancer results.

What Can You Actually Do?

So can we help this most important repair mechanism correct mismatches between *problems* and *correction resources*? Based on all the preceding information, here are some major considerations.

If there is a chance that your supply of mismatch repair genes will eventually run low, you can forestall that problem (or attack it from the other direction) by decreasing the demand. One of the simplest and most fundamental ways to do that is to limit your exposure to DNA damaging agents. And one of the best ways to do that is to cut down on or eliminate cigarettes, excessive alcohol, radiation, and chemically laden, processed junk foods, to name just a few potential instability-causing agents.

But can anything be done once some damage has occurred and genetic instability begins to set in? Researchers at Thomas Jefferson University's Jefferson Medical College and the University of Regensburg, Germany, believe they've uncovered a molecular mechanism that interferes with the genetic instability that increases the risk of colorectal cancer.[5] In other words, there is a substance that induces restoration of genetic stability: aspirin.

According to Richard Fishel, PhD, of Thomas Jefferson University in Philadelphia, common aspirin may prevent the development of a particular type of common hereditary colorectal cancer in those at high risk for the disease.[6]

Aspirin suppresses the accumulation of cancer-causing mutations in genetically unstable cells.*

In addition, certain nutrients specifically support DNA repair mechanisms—especially folate, often known by its more common name, folic acid. It's a B vitamin that is crucial to DNA synthesis and repair. People who don't get enough folate in their diets and who have inherited or acquired genetic instability are at a much greater risk of developing cancer.[7]

Individuals susceptible to genetic damage who don't get enough folate in their diet are almost three times as likely to develop bladder cancer as are those who eat plenty of fruits and vegetables and therefore have sufficient capacity to repair randomly occurring DNA damage. The ability to fix errant changes in DNA is of critical importance in maintaining normal genetic structure, and this ability is related to folate and other vitamins.

What's the overall message here? What we take into our bodies, especially certain foods, could provide one of the arrows that can strike at cancer's Achilles' heel. In section two, you will read about foods with the potential for amazing healing powers. But first, let me introduce you to an ominous concept—the immortality of cancer.

---

* Note: For various medical reasons, some people should not take aspirin, so please consult your personal health-care provider before consuming any food, supplement, or drug product.

Chapter 3

THE IMMORTAL CELL

I (Francisco Contreras) was born into a family of doctors and preachers. My father and my brother were both MDs, and all four of the men who married my sisters were ministers. I suppose I could have gamed the system by earning a doctor of divinity degree, but I followed in my father's footsteps and became an MD instead.

In earlier times, such career decisions were often made before the child was born, and in many parts of Europe they still are. Here in the New World, young men and women who follow their mothers and fathers into the "family business" are not the least bit unusual, even in our modern, do-your-own-thing age. I am extremely happy with the career I chose, but the point is that I *did* have a choice.

The Cell That Keeps on Living

The cells in your body do not have any such options. Granted, the nucleus of every cell contains a complete copy of your personal genome. Each of your brain cells, for example, has a complete set of the genetic blueprints necessary to build your liver, hands, hair, and eyes. Yet your brain cells produce only brain cells.

How and why cell differentiation happens is not yet fully understood. But clearly, even as fathers once absolutely decreed what their sons would do for a living before they were born, before any person is born certain built-in regulatory mechanisms precommit certain "cell lines" to develop a particular kind of tissue, without deviation.

This incredible (and equally essential) selectivity is achieved by complex regulatory mechanisms that turn on only the related genes while turning off all the rest. However, genes are also turned on or off by external factors such as contact inhibition, a mechanism that limits growth by respecting the surrounding tissues. (For example, even though the stomach is touching the liver, it never invades it.)

One of the most important regulatory mechanisms (if not the most important) that helps your body achieve controlled, functional, and harmonious development is the one that determines the life term of cells. In 1961, Dr. Leonard Hayflick discovered that there is a limit to how long a cell line can survive in a laboratory dish. In general, most cell lines age and die after about fifty divisions. This limitation is now called the Hayflick limit; it's a kind of retirement program in which old cells must die to give way to new recruits to continue function.

For the good of the whole body, this programmed cell life span is genetically predetermined, except for cells that are in charge of transferring information to other human beings via the normal human process of procreation through conception and birth. Thus, embryonic stem cells such as those from a fertilized human egg are immortal.

Literally, they have the power to develop into all of the 210 different kinds of cells in the body. Unfortunately, cancer cells are immortal too, as illustrated by the following story.

HeLa Cells

In the early 1950s, most pathologists, bound by convention and tradition, labeled a biopsy with carcinoma only if invasion could be documented as having already occurred. Yet some pathologists argued that cancer actually started before the malignant cells invaded other tissues. This revolutionary but logical concept, called carcinoma in situ (CIS), was first proposed by Dr. Richard W. Telinde from a Baltimore clinic, who found noninvasive malignant cells in the cervix of one of his patients, Henrietta Lacks, in 1951.

The controversy over whether to call it cancer, depending on whether the malignant cells have invaded other tissues, is still alive today. Likewise with respect to the cells from Henrietta Lacks's cervical cancer.

Mrs. Lacks's cells, to the surprise of Dr. Telinde, ignored the Hayflick limit and never stopped growing. These "immortal cells" are now known as HeLa cells in her memory. They continue to be cultured in laboratories around the world for research even today, more than fifty years later.[1]

The Telomere-Telomerase Connection

One of the crucial features that distinguishes a cancer cell from a normal cell is its ability to divide indefinitely. I'm about to use a few scientific terms, but bear with me.

A normal cell divides about fifty times and then dies—a process called *cellular senescence*. Regulation of this growth and development, of utmost importance so that our noses, feet, or ears will not grow to monstrous proportions, is the task of *telomeres*, which are protective buffers blocking the ends of chromosomes. The life cycle of each cell is determined by the length of its associated telomeres. With each cell division, the telomeres shorten so that at the last cell replication the telomere disappears, and the cell cannot make any other daughter cells and dies.

Two types of cells that are exempt from a predetermined life span are (1) gonadal cells, such as the ovum and the sperm, which must retain their ability to divide indefinitely from generation to generation without alteration, and (2) cancer cells. Cells of both of these types bypass the death cycle by stabilizing their telomeres via the action of an enzyme called *telomerase*, which in humans normally ceases after birth.

But cancer cells defy all this and turn on the genes responsible for telomerase production, resulting in stabilized telomere length. This is the trait of immortal cells.

Chinese researchers have shown that abnormal telomerase genes can be detected in about 90 percent of human tumors, while in surrounding healthier tissue the positive incidence of these genes was only about 3 percent.[2] Telomerase genes were overwhelmingly displayed in cancers of the breast, colon, gallbladder, lung, stomach, and esophagus,[3] as well as many other malignancies.[4]

As you might imagine, suppressing telomerase has been at the top of the lists of priorities of academic research facilities and many pharmaceutical giants all over the world for years. Indeed, scientists from the University of California–San Diego (UCSD) School of Medicine and Cancer Center, in collaboration with the Institute Pasteur in Paris, have developed a vaccine that specifically targets and destroys the telomerase proliferative peptide common to immortal cells.[5] No word yet on when the vaccine will be ready.

The development of therapies based on the promise of telomerase began in 1985. Human clinical trials with telomerase-inhibiting drugs didn't get underway in 2003. Geron, a pharmaceutical company, and Memorial-Sloan Kettering Cancer Center in New York received a joint grant from the National Cancer Institute to do the study. But again, when these drugs will be available to a cancer patient only our Lord knows. The latest headline is that the "telomerase breakthrough is not yet delivering the goods," according to a report of Geron (October 06, 2009), the company developing the vaccine. Geron continues its research and is featured at cancer research conferences as an absolute expert.[6] We are cheering the company on but not sitting on our hands. Our patients need help now.

The good news is that our cancer patients do *not* have to wait, for there are potential telomerase-inhibiting therapies available right now. Prescription drugs are not the only option for neutralizing telomerase. Over-the-counter drugs known as *nonsteroidal anti-inflammatory drugs* (NSAIDs), like indomethacin and ibuprofen, can bring about a dose-dependent reduction in telomerase activity.

Also, Japanese researchers have observed that high-dose green tea extract, available as a dietary supplement, could help cancer patients. Epigallocatechin gallate (EGCG), a fraction of green tea extract, has shown strong and direct telomerase-inhibiting effects. A dosage of five 350-mg capsules of green tea extract with each meal is now recommended.

All these antioxidants, readily available in health food stores, can help to reduce telomerase activity, according to the Fred Hutchinson Cancer Research Center.[7]

Chapter 4

HOW CANCER FIGHTS

*C*HU *CH*U *CHU chu AH AH Ah ah CHU CH*U *CHU chu AH AH Ah ah.* This is the unmistakable warning that Jason is coming in another sequel to the original *Friday the 13th* movie. Jason's victims used every weapon known to man against him—guns, fire, swords, explosives. They could knock Jason down, but eventually he would get up again and pursue. Even when someone *killed* Jason, he would reappear in the next movie.

The good news is that if you get too scared, you can just turn off your television or walk out of the theater. Not so with cancer, whose resilience is unbelievable. That's why cancer can be such a nightmare.

As I (Francisco Contreras) have explained before, the development of cancer therapies has been extremely difficult because of cancer's genetic instability. But several drugs, called chemotherapies, are effective in destroying cancer cells. Alas, in the process they also kill many of the good cells, causing all the dreaded side effects, while undermining the immune system.

Most of this damage is temporary, and our bodies are capable of restoration. But even the permanent damages caused by chemotherapy would be "acceptable"—when the patient can survive them—if the therapy would result in a cure or, at the very least, where the ratio of risk/benefit would be in favor of the patient. Statistically, the risk/benefit ratio, so far, is most certainly not in favor of most cancer patients.

At Oasis of Hope we have made great progress in protecting healthy cells from the devastation of chemotherapy. We are encouraged as we find new ways to overcome the failures of chemotherapy. We fully acknowledge, however, that chemotherapy is not a stand-alone treatment. It can only be a small part of a plan to beat cancer. Genetic profiling of each patient's cancer may, in the future, provide data as to which chemotherapy will work with a patient and which one will not. But right now, chemotherapy continues to be a hit-or-miss treatment.

Continuing Frustration

I almost cannot tell you how frustrating it is to watch a tumor disappear, only to see it come back, stronger than before, because the same chemotherapy that just "defeated" it would now be completely useless if used again. This process results in *resistance to chemotherapy*. In effect, cancer cells develop a shield, a "bulletproof vest" that protects them against that specific chemotherapy. At that point, only "second line" or even "third line" chemotherapy, usually with much less chance of success and necessarily much more aggressive, can be tried.

When the initial success lasts only a short time, patients who suffered through the tremendous side effects of "first line" chemotherapy are typically not so sure that suffering through another round of the same (or worse) thing is really worthwhile. Understandably, their frustration and their lack of confidence tend to be much deeper the second time around.

Meanwhile, to diminish resistance to the anticancer drugs, doctors often give an additional combination of *other* drugs. Unfortunately this has not solved the problem. In fact, if a cancer becomes resistant to one drug or one group of drugs, it often becomes resistant to other drugs, even when it has not been exposed to them. This is why it is very important to select the best possible treatment protocol, the so-called "first line" chemotherapies.

We are not sure why resistance develops, but it is attributed largely to cancer's capacity to adapt by using the cell's built-in intelligence and memory. Here are some of the current theories put forth to try to explain cell resistance:

- *Chemotherapy detoxification*: Cancer cells may pump the drug out of the cell as fast as it goes in using a molecule called p-glycoprotein.

- *Chemotherapy barrier*: Cancer cells may stop taking in the drugs because the protein that transports the drug across the cell wall stops working.

- *Chemotherapy neutralization*: Cancer cells may develop a mechanism that inactivates the drug.

- *Forced mutation*: The malignant cells that manage to survive chemotherapy mutate and become resistant to the drug.

- *Gene amplification*: Chemotherapy may trigger hundreds of copies of a particular gene, which in turn triggers an overproduction of protein that renders the anticancer drug ineffective.

- *DNA counter-repair*: The cancer cells may learn how to repair the DNA breaks caused by some anticancer drugs.

- *Aberrant DNA methylation*: In this metabolic process, the wrong genes are turned on to resist therapeutic agents.

Preventing and reducing resistance to chemotherapy in the treatment of cancer is a major research priority worldwide.

Fearfully and Wonderfully Made

More than twenty-five hundred years ago King David stated that our bodies were "fearfully and wonderfully made" (Ps. 139:14, NIV). Indeed, the more we find out about the intricacies of our bodies, the more wonders we admire. One of those most amazing wonders is that every one of your body's 100 trillion cells carries your body's entire genomic information.

How is it, then, that if every cell has the blueprint for your whole system, liver cells produce only liver cells? The short answer is that liver cells turn on only the genes necessary to produce liver cells and turn off every other gene. Cells constantly have to make choices—for example, once they choose the cell line, they also have to turn on the right genes to produce specific substances, such as hormones or enzymes, according to the body's needs. This is what we call the cell's intelligence.

But how does the cell "decide" to activate and deactivate genes? The *most nearly understood process* is called DNA methylation.

This is a complicated chemical process, but let me give you the best simplified explanation we have. Methylation is the passing of a chemical—belonging to the methyl group—from one molecule to another. This methyl group acts as a "tag" that signals some of the most important metabolic functions throughout our bodies.[1]

Unfortunately, there is good and bad DNA methylation. Here are just a few of the many examples of the good. Methylation is used to make:

- Melatonin (the sleep hormone)
- Adrenaline (the fight-or-flight hormone)
- Acetylcholine (a neurotransmitter)
- Creatine (for muscle energy metabolism)
- Carnitine (involved in fat burning in mitochondria)
- Choline (fat mobilization and cell membrane fluidity)

The consequences of bad or aberrant DNA methylation include silencing of tumor-suppressor-gene expression.[2] In simpler English, this might be somewhat like turning all the traffic signals in New York City to green at the same time. No one would know when and where to stop, and the results would be horrific.[3]

But getting back to our subject, aberrant DNA methylation can switch on or off the genes that can turn the once-useful chemicals in a course of chemotherapy into substances that, for all the good they can do you, might as well be inert.

Professor Robert Brown at Glasgow University, in Scotland, is using a drug called decitabine in clinical studies for the treatment of advanced myelodysplastic syndrome because of its unique mechanism of action and its regulation of DNA methylation. Thus recent advances in the way we study DNA methylation in the human genome are uncovering many important genes that may be targets for chemotherapy.[4]

While some positive clinical results with drugs that undo bad DNA methylation have been reported—like the one Professor Brown is proposing—it's likely to be many years (or decades) before this new breed of drugs will be available to patients. Decitabine, a DNA methyltransferase inhibitor, is still in animal studies, but we are keeping our eyes on this type of research because it shows so much promise.[5]

Fortunately, we do not have to wait for these drugs. Understanding the metabolic methylation pathways of nutrition is imperative for developing strategies to prevent methylation-related problems, such as chronic diseases, carcinogenesis, and chemo-resistance. The evidence suggests that folate, which mediates methyl-group transfers, is critical for ensuring the integrity of biological methylation and for maintaining the proper pathways needed to maintain normal DNA metabolism.[6] That's another reason why I recommended, at the end of chapter 2, that you increase your intake of folate.

Hopefully this chapter has increased your understanding of how cancer fights to stay alive. This foundation will help you as you read the next chapter, where I discuss the three main cancer-fighting weapons of conventional medicine.

Chapter 5

THE THREE MAJOR WEAPONS OF CONVENTIONAL MEDICINE

A LITTLE MORE THAN TWENTY YEARS AGO, A FRIEND NAMED Richard called me (Francisco Contreras) to share some exciting news. He'd just bought a beach house at a terrific price, just south of Rosarito on the picturesque coastline of Baja, California. He invited my wife and me to come down to enjoy a nice weekend.

When we arrived, I instantly figured out why he'd gotten such a smoking deal. His new place was the worst fixer-upper I had ever seen! The roof leaked so badly you could get a spotted suntan from indoors. But we survived that first visit, and over the next few years we watched Rich put so much money into the house that he should have changed his first name to Poor. Dry rot, rusted pipes, you name it—everything was falling apart.

In 1984, a huge storm pounded the coastline and swept hundreds of homes and businesses away. I hoped that my friend's problems would be solved by nature, but that disaster of a house somehow survived!

The search for a cure for cancer reminds me of the money-pit nature of Rich's house. Consider this quote: "Between 1970 and 1994, federal health expenditures grew from $18 billion to $328 billion, about a 1700 percent gain."[1] What have hundreds of billions of dollars, over the last forty years, produced so far?

Well, we still have the same options we had forty years ago: chemotherapy, radiation, and surgery. Granted, techniques and equipment are more sophisticated than ever, but they are basically the same. As the research dollars go up, you would expect the incidence and mortality rates to go down. Not so.

In 1971, there were 337,361 cancer deaths reported. In 2009, the toll was 562,340, according to the American Cancer Society's (ACS) annual cancer statistics report, "Cancer Facts & Figures 2009."[2] In this report it is also mentioned that cancer death rates are minimally but steadily falling (1.8 percent a year among men from 2001–2005 and 0.6 percent a year from 1998–2005 among women). They credit the improvement to, in large part, better prevention, increased use of early detection practices, and improved treatments for cancer.

These results are challenged by the "World Cancer Report" of the International Agency for Research on Cancer (IARC), published December 10, 2008.[3] In this report they state, "Cases of cancer doubled globally between 1975 and 2000," and predict that cancers diagnosed "will double again by 2020, and will nearly triple by 2030. There were an estimated 12 million new cancer diagnoses and more than 7 million deaths worldwide [in 2008]. The projected numbers for 2030 are 20 to 26 million new diagnoses and 13 to 17 million deaths." It is interesting that all this is directly related to the Americanization of the world. The increase of diabetes and cancer parallel the global explosion of the US junk-food industry.

A deeper look into the ACS's 2009 report on cancer improvement trends puts their numbers in doubt. First, most epidemiologists credit the results to the diminishing smoking habits of Americans as the most likely cause, not early detection or intervention. The ACS's chief executive officer, John R. Seffrin, PhD, seems to agree. On December 9, 2008, in Atlanta, Georgia, the leading US cancer organizations met to unite against the *global cancer burden* in lieu of the before-mentioned IARC's report. Seffrin's comment at that meeting was, "For all of our ninety-five years the Society has pursued the vow of our founders to eliminate cancer in all humankind. We recognize that cancer strikes without regard to borders or socioeconomic status, and we support cancer control initiatives in more than twenty countries, and fund capacity building and tobacco control grants in some seventy countries—including the launch next week of our tobacco Quitline in India. It is my hope that by bringing proven interventions to places in the world impacted most by this disease, we can diminish needless suffering and save many lives."[4] He clearly believes that an anti-tobacco campaign is the most effective cancer damage control action and that in its ninety-five years, the ACS has little more to report on the advances of cancer control.

Secondly, the cancer death toll has risen from 337,361 in 1971 to 562,340 in 2009. This is a 74 percent increase, while the population has increased only by 51 percent. More so, in this period (1970–2009) a great percentage of the population's increase is due to immigration (1986 mass amnesty) from countries such as Mexico, with much lower incidences and death rates from cancer that very well might have "diluted" the American cancer death toll mentioned by the ACS's "Cancer Facts & Figures 2009" reports of the last few years.

You would be justified to suggest that conventional therapies have been a qualified failure.

But hold on a moment. Before we write off conventional therapies altogether, let's take a look at history, and let's see where we are going in the future. For every person who is uncomfortable when I recommend conventional therapies, I know another person who is equally opposed to alternative therapies. Perhaps the following paragraphs will help these people—and you as well—understand when and why I would opt for conventional treatments and when and why I would not.

Chemotherapy

The first precept of pharmacology 101 is that *all medications have the potential to cure the disease for which they were designed, but they also have the potential to kill the patient.* Thus it is of utmost importance to understand the mechanisms by which they act and their dosages.

Chemotherapy is no exception to this time-honored rule. Even though this very aggressive therapy, in general, often causes more harm than good, we must never underestimate its potential for good if it is properly applied when precisely indicated.

I—and many others—have often been a severe critic of chemotherapy because of its poor track record. Nonetheless, very few medications by themselves are purely good or purely bad. What typically determine the outcome are the criteria of the therapist. I believe that chemotherapy has a bad rap due to its excessive and forceful indications. In other words, oncologists prescribe it in high dosages and multiple combinations for poor candidates, patients who really are not going to benefit, especially in the long run. I will explain our criteria for chemotherapy use at the Oasis of Hope Hospital,[5] but first I must qualify my criticism.

A very revealing summary of the results of chemotherapy was published by Dr. Ulrich Abel in *Chemotherapy for Advanced Epithelial Cancer*, in which he erects one of the most solid pillars of orthodox oncology.[6] The term *epithelial cancer* encompasses cancer of the lungs, breast, prostate, colon, and other organs. Epithelial cancers are responsible for 80 percent of the deaths attributable to cancer in the industrialized world. During his ten years as a statistician, Abel discovered that the method used for treating the most commonly occurring epithelial cancers has rarely been successful.

Such a judgment is significant when we consider that Dr. Abel stated that an "almost dogmatic belief in the efficacy of chemotherapy is usually based on false conclusions from inaccurate data."[7] An article in the *Journal of Clinical Oncology* revealed that, in a survey involving 118 doctors and many cancer specialists in Canada, the following question was posed: "Were you to develop inoperable lung cancer, would you be willing to receive mandated doses of multi-chemotherapy?" The vast majority emphatically answered no.[8]

Please let me remind you, chemotherapy is a tool available at Oasis of Hope. But it cannot be used blindly. For it to be effective and not destroy the quality of the patient's life, it must be used in conjunction with a comprehensive support program.

Let me clarify further. In 1986, Dr. J. C. Bailar III and Elaine Smith reported that patients with lung cancer who were not treated have a longer life expectancy and enjoy a better quality of life than those who receive treatment.[9] In 1988, Dr. Abel reported that in an experiment with patients suffering from pancreatic cancer, those who received the placebo treatment instead of the real treatment lived longer and better.[10]

These two studies demonstrate that chemotherapy cannot work without supporting therapies like the ones we have integrated into our treatment program at Oasis of Hope. Our patients who take chemotherapy as a part of their overall treatment program outlive and beat all of the statistics.

Dr. Bailar, upon evaluating the results of cancer therapies between 1950 and 1982, concluded that mortality due to cancer continued to increase. And in 1986, he professed that "35 years of intense effort focused largely on improving treatment must be judged a qualified failure."[11] Eleven years later (in 1997), a reevaluation published in the *New England Journal of Medicine* reported that the mortality rate for people with cancer continued to climb.[12] Oncologists really need to look beyond neutralizing the tumor with chemotherapy. That is why our focus is on treating the whole patient with as many natural interventions as possible and using chemotherapy in new and innovative ways that are effective with few side effects.

Chemotherapy has its merits and indications. *The second basic precept of pharmacology is that the difference between a cure and a poison is the dosage.* Even the most natural and nontoxic agent, given inappropriately, can kill a patient. By the same token, in appropriate dosages even chemotherapy can help a patient.

Radiation

Radiation therapy is the second line of attack. For a short time, total body radiation was used; however, that was stopped when many patients died from extreme toxicity. Now radiation therapy has evolved into a localized therapy in which dosages, as well as the size of the fields (the areas where the radiation is beamed), have diminished significantly.

X-ray-type beams are used to burn malignant cells. Still, some patients have adverse reactions to the therapy because, even though the fields are limited, within the field the beam will still go through benign as well as malignant cells.

In my opinion radiation therapy, in which we placed so much faith a few decades ago, has proven to be beneficial in very few cases. Side effects of this therapy include severe nausea, malaise, loss of appetite, and the loss of other functions.

Radiation doses have to be specifically measured, and there is an air dose, a skin dose, and a tumor dose. The calculation has to be done by an expert, many times by a physicist. The radiation therapist does the planning to prevent the burning of the skin. The lighter the skin, the more it will be affected.

Each phase has to be analyzed and individualized to see if there are overriding benefits to the patients. As the Europeans say, "Why should we *cause* symptoms when the patient doesn't *have* any symptoms?"

Fortunately, new technology is now available that concentrates radiation to the tumor, which significantly reduces radiation to skin and other organs. This is achieved by radiating the tumor from many different angles. In cases where bone is being destroyed by cancer, either in primary cancer of the bones or when cancer has spread to the bones, the value of radiation is immense. Cancer in the bones can be very painful, and radiation is incredibly effective at controlling the pain and hardening the bones to help avoid fractures. But the merits of radiation are limited to only a few types of cancer.

Surgery

We have already discovered that much of conventional cancer therapy is based on the theory that tumors are the disease and should be destroyed. There are several ways to remove or destroy invasive, malignant clusters of cells. The most primitive is surgery.

Literally hundreds of procedures have been developed to remove tumors from all parts of the anatomy. Tumors may be so large and in such "inconvenient" parts of the body (perhaps dangerously close to—or even overlaying—a vital organ) that often a surgeon must come up with an individual technique to remove a specific tumor without endangering the patient. This is my specialty, and it is challenging.

Sometimes there is little that surgery can offer. At other times, surgeries lasting twelve or more hours can remove complicated tumors, thus granting the patient his best chance of recovery. Even so, believe it or not, surgery is the least aggressive of the orthodox treatments.

Surgery can be a helpful and compassionate cancer treatment. If one of my patients has an obstructed intestinal track, I would not give him carrots to eat or tell him that juicing those carrots will cure him. They might even kill him. In his case, surgery would be a lifesaver.

I am alarmed, however, at how aggressive some surgeons have become. We need to be conservative about when and how we suggest a surgery. Any type of surgery is stressful on a patient and involves risks.

Consider surgery in breast cancer patients. For years, radical mastectomies were the only option. The whole breast, the surrounding lymph nodes, and sometimes even the pectoral muscle were removed. Why was surgery so aggressive? Because of a belief that cancer only spreads through extension. The goal was to cut out as much tissue surrounding the tumor as possible to try to get any "likely extension" of it. But then we learned that cancer can spread through the bloodstream, and that removing huge portions of tumor-surrounding tissue does not improve the prognosis of the patient. All it does is decrease that patient's quality of life.

Now many surgeries are offering to remove the tumor only, which is called a lumpectomy. I have been convinced by reviewing clinical studies and through personal experience that, in general, lumpectomies are as effective as radical mastectomies. Plus, they leave the woman's body intact, which is very important to the patient.

It is true that 20 percent of the patients treated with conservative surgery (lumpectomy) experience recurrences, but it is also true that they can be treated with another conservative operation. Although 20 percent seems like a high percentage, remember that 80 percent are spared a devastating operation that would severely reduce the quality of their lives. Vera Peter, MD, of Toronto considered that "although the rate of recurrence is significantly higher in patients treated with conservative surgery, their life expectancy is the same."[13]

In 1985 the National Surgical Adjuvant Breast Project (NSABP) published the first results of a comparative study of conservative surgical treatments (simple mastectomy and lumpectomy with postoperative radiation therapy). The study concluded that patients treated with a lumpectomy, the most conservative treatment, lived as long as those who received one of the other treatments.

Radical surgery is still, incredibly, the favored approach for the treatment of breast cancer. Nevertheless, this approach is slowly being modified even as the conservative approach is gaining acceptance.

Am I against surgery? Absolutely not. I am a surgical oncologist. That means that as a cancer doctor, my specialty is surgery. What I am against is being unnecessarily aggressive in surgery. I remember a twenty-something young mother who came to Oasis of Hope literally running away from surgery. She had a tumor behind her knee the size of a basketball, and her oncologist recommended amputation of her entire leg, up through the hip. After reviewing her X-rays, I concluded that we could remove the tumor without amputating the leg, though it would be a long, arduous, and delicate surgery. We then gave her an integrative therapy to reduce the risk of recurrence, which in this case is high; thus the "need" for the amputation. It gave me great joy to see this woman walk out of the hospital on her own power, holding her son's hand. Because of our multipronged approach, the patient is still alive and enjoying the use of her leg after more than fifteen years.

Why Are These Three Methods Not Enough?

The failures of conventional therapies do not result from the procedures themselves but from how and why they are used. This is true for two primary reasons.

1. Based on a false premise

First, their application is based on a false premise, that *cancerous tumors are the disease*. In reality, the tumors are but symptoms of the metabolic failures that allowed them to grow.

Thus, removing or destroying tumors is only a half-measure. Our failure to restore the organic deficiencies that caused the tumors in the first place is what accounts for most cancer recurrences and deaths.

And yet, success is often still measured by what happens to the tumor, not by what happens to the patient.

2. The criteria with which they are offered

The second reason for failure is the criteria with which chemotherapy, radiation, and surgery are offered. If the cancer is aggressive, the therapy must be aggressive. Maximum tumor mass must be removed or radiated, as much as the patient can tolerate, and chemotherapy will be given.

Sadly, when it is understood that the disease is much more than the tumor, all of these procedures, in limited cases, can diminish tumor mass. My first criterion for using them is whether I would be willing to be on the receiving end if I were my own patient. My second criterion is whether that procedure is likely to improve the patient's quality of life.

Asking myself these questions keeps me motivated to find effective, non-harmful ways to help my patients. I am very enthusiastic about how much information is coming to the surface as many researchers are finding how natural therapies can overcome the shortfalls of conventional therapy. In fact, we have used this information effectively to the point where most of my patients will now receive chemotherapy, yes, even at Oasis of Hope. Oasis of Hope was the one place where patients could go to escape chemotherapy, and our shift over the last ten years has left people scratching their heads.

I find myself many times between a rock and a hard place. On the one hand, I'm criticized by the alternative doctors for offering conventional therapies. On the other hand, I have been chastised by oncologists for administering alternative therapies to my patients. "So which is it, orthodox or alternative medicine?" they ask. In truth, I am not phased by these reproaches. What type of medicine do I adhere to? Whatever medicine is best for my patient. For me there is not "either/or" but an integration of both to better combat cancer.

I mentioned before that the foundation for achieving a goal is a proper philosophy. My father established a treatment philosophy based on two principles: 1) do no harm, and 2) love your patient as you love yourself.

How then can the use of harmful chemotherapy and radiation be administered at the Oasis of Hope? Are we offering therapeutic protocols that we ourselves would take if faced with cancer? The answer is a resounding yes! By integrating and regulating conventional and alternative therapies, a concept we christened integrative regulatory therapies, we have not only significantly reduced the negative side effects of chemotherapy and radiation therapy, but we have also significantly increased their efficacy. If you ever come to Oasis of Hope, know that we will look at every aspect of your specific needs, and we will tailor a treatment program that will best position your body to heal itself. This may or may not include chemotherapy, radiation, or surgery. But when we use these interventions, we are nonaggressive, and they only form about 15 percent of the overall treatment program. Conventional therapies don't cure cancer. They can be beneficial and helpful to kill cancer cells, but they should only be a small part of the overall healing process. So how can they be used effectively?

This is achieved by a multipronged protective "umbrella" that maintains the integrity and function of healthy cells through oxidative preconditioning, oxygenation of tumors, signaling transduction, immune stimulation, diet, and emotional and spiritual support. Our focus on quality of life, versus tumor destruction, is one of the main reasons why so many of our patients are doing well.

I must mention that there are many cases in which chemotherapy and radiation therapy are not the best antitumor therapies. This is what is so exciting about Oasis of Hope. We have many other therapies to offer

SECTION II
TWENTY WAYS TO BEAT CANCER

MODERN DOCTORS OFTEN DEFINE *HEALTH* AS "THE ABSENCE OF illness." Hippocrates defined *health* as "the perfect balance between man and his environment."

To modify the words of Hippocrates, it could be said that optimal health resides in a perfect balance between the Creator and His creation. But before man can achieve that optimal balance with God, he first needs to achieve a healthy balance among his own body, mind, and spirit.

Spiritual health means many things to many people. Often the word *religion* gets treated like a four-letter word. The "in" thing now is to say, "I'm not religious, but I am very spiritual." Either way, the important question is, How can you cultivate a healthy spirit?

Part of the answer comes when you learn to recognize the symptoms of a spirit in distress versus a spirit in balance. Some of the products of a healthy spirit are love, joy, peace, perseverance, gentleness, goodness, humility, and self-control. The signs of a spirit in distress include anger, resentment, hatred, bitterness, excessive worry, and the ultimate spiritual stronghold of cancer—fear.

In section two the discussion turns to the main strategies for fighting cancer. Some of them are purely physical, like taking a walk or changing your diet; some are emotional—forgiveness, for instance, or a hopeful mind-set; and some are spiritual.

Just as there is no such thing as an atheist in a foxhole, so there is rarely such a thing as an atheist in a cancer ward. Cancer has a way of showing us very quickly just where our own powers end. And yet there, at that place where your power ceases, the power of God's Spirit begins.

Chapter 6

CONSIDER THESE ALTERNATIVE THERAPIES

Cancer Beaters #1–4

NOW THAT WE'VE COVERED THE BASICS ABOUT CANCER AND the three main conventional approaches to fighting it, we'd like to let you know about some lesser-known approaches that we have used at Oasis of Hope for years to help overcome the deficiencies of chemotherapy, radiation, and surgery. Read about them and then decide whether you'd like to have access to this type of eclectic cancer treatment or stick with the basics. The procedures are ozone therapy, hyperbaric oxygen therapy, ultraviolet light therapy, melatonin therapy, and one of the latest advances at Oasis of Hope—lymphocyte therapy.

Cancer Beater #1:
Ozone Therapy

When most people hear the word *ozone*, they think of what they often smell after a thunderstorm, when lightning has literally "supercharged" the air. Or, if they remember their high school science class, they think of the ozone layer as an invisible but protective "blanket" near (or at) the top of our atmosphere.

In nature, however, ozone has both a good side and a bad side. High up in the stratosphere it acts as a shield, deflecting harmful UV irradiation.

However, a little lower down in the troposphere, ozone is a major component of the smog that harms humans, animals, and plants. When we breathe it, even though it can feel like a tonic in small concentrations, ozone can cause serious pulmonary and systemic side effects.

Ozone itself is nothing more than oxygen with a molecular structure of O_3 instead of O_2. The numbers indicate how many atoms make up each molecule; thus, the "supercharged" concept is not a bad analogy.

However, the additional atom in each molecule makes ozone a highly reactive oxidant. Imagine a carbon steel knife blade left to rust on a bench. If the bench were in your garage, the knife blade might be completely covered by rust in several months. But if the same knife were sealed into an ozone-rich atmosphere, the same result might be achieved in a matter of days.

However, one particular anticancer application of ozone is very therapeutic.

It has been shown that ozone supports broad-spectrum antimicrobial activity. This means that it fights the bacteria that cause infection. In the First World War, medics used it to save the lives of wounded soldiers suffering from gaseous gangrene. Today, ozonated solutions and ozonated oils are still used to treat wounds and a host of infections. Ozone therapies are used to treat fistulae, abscesses, ulcers, gingivitis, stomatitis, and osteomyelitis.

Ozone therapy became an alternative medical approach in 1954, when Wehrly and Steinbart first described its application.[1] They found that while the human respiratory tract reacts very negatively to ozone, human blood does not. In fact, when exposed to appropriate ozone concentrations, our blood antioxidant capacity counteracts the strong oxidant properties of ozone, thus eliminating any acute side effects.

The benefits derived from this therapy are staggering. For example, Oasis doctors know that ozonation of the blood improves the exchange of oxygen in the blood, activates the immune system, and increases the efficiency of the antioxidant system. But what is most exciting to us is how these three activities combine to effectively retard or reverse tumor growth.

Over the last seventeen years, doctors at Oasis have advanced the use of ozone therapy, and the results have been extraordinary. Our patients have experienced measurable tumor reduction quickly, sometimes in as little as two weeks. For long-term results, we still believe that slower-acting metabolic therapy is vital, but it is wonderful to get fast results, too.[2] Indeed, ozone provokes a cascade of effects when it is introduced into the bloodstream.

How does ozone therapy work?

This section gets a bit technical, but we've put it here because it's so fundamental to our understanding.

Ozone decomposes in blood and interacts immediately with several substances: fatty acids, cholesterols, proteins, and carbohydrates. When the ozone decomposes, a series of reactive oxygen species are quickly produced, the most important of which is hydrogen peroxide (H_2O_2).

A sudden rise in H_2O_2 concentration triggers very different biochemical activity depending upon the type of cell the H_2O_2 penetrates. If the H_2O_2 penetrates red cells and endothelial cells, three things happen.

- First, there is an increase in the delivery and release of oxygen by red cells toward the tissues, especially hypoxic tumor areas.

- Second, in areas of the system that were constricted, endothelial cells enhance release of nitric oxide (NO), resulting in dilation of blood vessels and improving oxygen flow.

- Third, the formation of new blood vessels (angiogenesis) is inhibited due to improved oxygenation in the neoplastic tissue.

Ozone is an oxidant and provokes a natural antioxidant effect that prepares the body for oxidant therapies and reduces the side effects of chemotherapy and radiation therapy. The oxidation also unleashes a beneficial immune chain reaction in favor of the patient.

These effects can be achieved by ozone or by breathing pure oxygen while in a pressurized chamber. This is called hyperbaric oxygen therapy, sometimes abbreviated HBO or HBOT. (*Hyper* means "over" and *baric* refers to atmospheric pressure.) Hyperbaric oxygen has actually been in use in a primitive form since the 1600s. However, modern HBOT was developed by the military after World War I to treat divers with decompression sickness. The work was expanded after World War II, and clinical trials during the 1950s revealed a number of beneficial mechanisms from HBOT.

The basis of HBOT is a law of physics called Henry's Law, which states, "The solubility of a gas in a liquid is directly proportional to the pressure of that gas above the surface of the solution." What this means in practical terms is that when a person is put in a sealed chamber filled with oxygen, and the pressure of the chamber is increased, then the oxygen will dissolve in the body's blood and other body fluids; the higher the pressure, the more oxygen will be dissolved. This makes it possible to perfuse the body with oxygen in increased amounts and have it carried to tissues that might not be accessible through normal respiration.

Part of the Oasis of Hope cancer treatment program in our center in Southern California is to give patients hyperbaric oxygen sessions of sixty to ninety minutes at a pressure of 2.5 atmospheres. We combine these sessions with nutraceuticals and a safe drug called Trental (pentoxifylline) to augment HBOT's effect. Trental is an FDA-approved drug used to improve the flow of blood by decreasing its viscosity (making it thinner), increasing blood flow to the microcirculation system and enhancing tissue oxygenation.

In recent years, more and more research is being conducted in the area of oxygen and hyperbaric oxygen that suggest it could be an important element in the treatment of cancer. One such study concluded that increasing the partial pressure of oxygen in tumors may in fact reduce the formation of new blood vessels, a process that is called angiogenesis. This can result in a significant slowing of tumor growth.[3]

Remember, tumors feed on blood vessels. Thus, anything that reduces the formation of blood vessels helps to restrain tumor growth.

When H_2O_2 penetrates cells known as leukocytes, it induces the production of specialized biological assassins called cytokines. These include interleukins, interferon, and tumor necrosis factor. The cytokines launch an array of immune functions, such as macrophages and neutrophils, which slow tumor growth and metastasis.

The presence of H_2O_2 in the blood increases the efficiency with which the body eliminates oxidants. We know that persistent oxidative stress from free radicals, or oxidants, is at the root of degenerative diseases such as cancer. Countless findings show that aging, chronic viral infections, cancer, autoimmune diseases, and neurodegenerative diseases are all accompanied by reductions in the body's ability to detoxify itself properly.

Without question, ozone therapy will rapidly become an essential tool for oncologists and an integral part of comprehensive treatment programs. Over the next few years, Oasis of Hope doctors will continue to refine its use, and I expect even more dramatic results.

Cancer Beater #2:
Ultraviolet Light

Researchers began to consider the use of ultraviolet light to treat disease in the 1870s. At that time, scientists understood that ultraviolet light was extremely efficient at eliminating bacteria. Dr. Niels Ryberg Finsen and several other prominent physicians of that era suggested using ultraviolet light to destroy infectious organisms in the blood. Finsen was one of the first researchers to irradiate blood with ultraviolet light. In 1903, he won the Nobel Prize in Medicine for his work in treating the blood of three hundred lupus patients with ultraviolet light.

The next major innovation in the therapy came in 1928, when

American researchers E. Knott and V. Hancock used a device that made extracorporeal ultraviolet blood irradiation (UVBI) possible. They conducted the first successful treatment of septic infection with the therapy. Later work revealed that ultraviolet light has a positive influence on the immune, respiratory, and hormonal systems.

So why has it been regarded as a new therapy? Sadly, the answer is all too clear. A host of new antibiotics and vaccines were introduced in the 1950s. The medical industry was so enthusiastic to use these products that the UVBI device went on the shelf. This is especially disappointing because for many illnesses, such as hepatitis and pneumonia, UVBI treatment was clearly superior. Thankfully, interest in UVBI therapy was rekindled two decades later in Russia.

How is the ultraviolet light treatment administered?

Two pieces of equipment are needed to administer extracorporeal UVBI therapy. The first, obviously, is a source of ultraviolet light. The second is an irradiation chamber made from quartz glass, which is permeable for ultraviolet radiation.

The standard procedure is known as the Knott technique,[4] which uses the following steps.

1. Doctors draw 1.5 ml of blood per pound of body weight, never exceeding 250 ml. The blood is drawn into a transfusion flask containing a small amount of an anticoagulant, such as heparin or citrate. This additive prevents clots from forming in the bottle or the tubing.

2. The blood is pumped through the special tubing at a controlled rate (approximately 0.5 ml/sec). The blood flows through an irradiation chamber, called a cuvette, where it is exposed for up to ten seconds to a controlled amount of ultraviolet irradiation in a therapeutic band, generated by specialized lamps.

3. When the correct amount of blood has been irradiated and stored in a flask, the flow is reversed and the blood is irradiated a second time as it returns to the body.

4. In addition to the "standard" three steps above, at the Oasis of Hope an extra step is added. Blood is ozonized just before reinfusion, because the combined effectiveness of the two therapies is greater than if they were administered separately.

The entire procedure takes thirty minutes. This includes ten minutes for setup and ten minutes for cleanup. The new devices at Oasis use disposable crystal reaction chambers and disposable tubing to avoid using potentially contaminated materials.

The treatment variables can be tailored to the needs of each patient. Some patients receive treatment daily; others, weekly. Some patients receive a course of three sessions; others as many as eight. Some patients treat 100 ml of blood each session; others up to 250 ml.

The best thing about the therapy is how it works. During the early years of UVBI therapy, Dr. E. K. Knott and his associates sought to explain how the treatment obtains its therapeutic effects. Research has identified two probable modes.

1. The first explanation is that the ultraviolet irradiation destroys bacteria and viruses in the extracted blood and creates a kind of "vaccination effect." In other words, when the irradiated blood returns to the body, the immune system identifies the dead bacteria and viruses in it. It then seeks out and destroys the same bacteria and viruses in the nonirradiated blood in the rest of the body.

2. The second explanation is that when the small fraction of irradiated blood is reinfused, it begins to spread throughout the entire volume of blood in the body. These

irradiated blood cells give off secondary radiation. The secondary radiation destroys viruses, bacteria, and toxins. In addition, it activates white blood cells.

Strong evidence suggests that UVBI therapy has a prophylactic action against cancer. A study in East Germany measured the number of mutations produced by chromosomes. After six sessions of UVBI therapy, researchers found that the number of chromosomal mutations diminished. These doctors believe that UVBI therapy can actually stimulate DNA repair.[5]

Compared to orthodox treatments, UVBI therapy is extremely safe. A Russian study of 2,380 sessions of UVBI therapy revealed that only 1.3 percent of patients experienced side effects and that the side effects were mild.[6] The potential benefits clearly outweigh the slight potential of mild side effects.

At Oasis of Hope Hospital we combine ozonation with UV irradiation of the blood. On one hand, irradiation of the blood begins the process of transforming monocytes into immature dendritic cells. On the other, it is known that oxidative stress generated during ozonation and UV irradiation of the blood, or HBOT, at the moment of reinfusion promotes maturation of dendritic cells.[7]

The mechanical stress to which the white blood cells (known as *monocytes*) are subjected during the procedure induces them to convert into dendritic antigen-presenting cells. These are the cells that initiate immune reactions by identifying targets for the immune system.[8]

Ultimately, the various applications of ultraviolet light as an antitumor agent are very exciting. My hope is that more and more cancer treatment facilities will incorporate emerging therapies such as UVBI and HBOT into their programs. These therapies are incredibly effective, and they do not destroy the immune system or compromise the emotional health of the patient.

Cancer Beater #3:
Melatonin

Another one of nature's wonders is a substance called melatonin. This neurohormone is synthesized and secreted at night by the pineal gland, which is located in the brain.[9]

Studies have found that melatonin is a highly effective antitumor agent. Melatonin does a number of important things. It inhibits the proliferation of cancer cells, stimulates mechanisms that fight cancer, encourages proper gene expression, and scavenges free radicals.[10]

Several clinical studies also provide strong evidence suggesting that melatonin can inhibit cancer cell growth. In one such study, melatonin was administered to 1,440 patients with "untreatable" tumors.[11] In another study, melatonin was given to 200 patients with chemotherapy-resistant tumors.[12] In both studies, the frequency of cachexia, asthenia, thrombocytopenia, and lymphocytopenia was significantly lower for patients treated with melatonin than the control group. Moreover, the percentage of patients with disease stabilization was significantly higher for patients treated with melatonin than in the control group. In other words, the melatonin appeared to slow or halt the development of existing tumors.

Other studies indicate that melatonin stimulates some of the mechanisms in the body that combat cancer. For example, studies show that melatonin amplifies the antitumoral activity of interleukin-2.[13] Scientists have also determined that a reduction in melatonin concentration can cause a deficiency in immune function.

One result of this is a reduction in tumor surveillance, the body's ability to recognize and combat tumor growth. The immune surveillance system plays a critical role in preventing cancer by recognizing the formation of abnormal cells. T cells in particular are valuable for their ability to distinguish mutated cells from normal cells. But when the immune system is suppressed, the mutated carcinoma cells are not recognized by the immune surveillance system, and the cells grow uncontrollably and become cancerous. When the body gets enough melatonin, the tumor surveillance system functions as it was designed to do.

For cells to reproduce properly, they have to be able to accurately receive genetic instructions. Studies show that melatonin increases the gap-junction-intercellular communication, in which area most cancer cells have some dysfunction. In addition, many tumor-promoting chemicals cause this dysfunction in intercellular communication, whereas chemicals like melatonin improve intercellular communication. The better the communication, the less likely a cell is to produce a cancer.

Remember what we said about genetic instability? Melatonin is an important natural agent that helps reduce mutations and DNA instability.

Finally, melatonin is one of the most powerful antioxidants found in nature. Research shows that it protects DNA, cell membranes, lipids, and proteins from free-radical damage. Another important quality of melatonin is its ability to enter all cells of the body and every subcellular compartment. This means that melatonin can enter a cell's nucleus and scavenge the free radicals responsible for DNA damage.

Since the radical-scavenging function of melatonin is dose-dependent, a decreased melatonin concentration is directly connected with a diminished protection of DNA, leading to a higher risk of cancer. Melatonin is a highly effective scavenger of the hydroxyl free radicals, which are considered the most damaging of all the free radicals.

Recently a study was published that concluded that patients with metastatic cancer of the lung or gastrointestinal tract who were administered melatonin experienced longer survival rates.[14] For all of these reasons, the administration of melatonin is a part of the Oasis of Hope program. We believe it is an important tool the body can use to ward off disease.

Cancer Beater #4:
Lymphocyte Therapy

Lymphocyte therapy is an exciting new therapy based on research by Dr. Kondo in Japan.[15] His work is focused on the allogeneic effect (an immune response due to foreign agent) in a cancer patient caused by the infusion of T lymphocytes from a young, healthy, unrelated donor.

Recently, researchers from Johns Hopkins University have discovered that this therapy activates dendritic cells and natural killer cells to destroy cancer cells.[16] (Dendritic cells, also called presenter cells, are part of the immune system designed to localize abnormal cells and "present" them to destroyer cells for annihilation.) We are very excited about the preliminary results being reported and see a great future for this type of natural immune system therapy.

There is also something amazing about how we use this therapy at Oasis of Hope. Our donors are not strangers off the street. They are Oasis of Hope staff members, and the patients are able to meet them. Patients are so grateful and touched that our team members not only give loving care, but they also literally give of themselves to help patients beat cancer.

Chapter 7

ADDRESS YOUR IMMUNE SYSTEM

Cancer Beater #5

I (FRANCISCO CONTRERAS) GREW UP ON JACQUES COUSTEAU'S underwater specials on TV. It didn't matter what Cousteau was saying; his French accent made it sound important. One night the show demonstrated the behavior of some type of stonefish that would bury itself in the sand with only its eyes poking out. Cousteau's narration went something like this: "Zee predeteur lies en wait unteel eh leetl unsuspecting crustazion gwuud trai to marche bai."

Provided this opportunity, the lethal stonefish struck at lighting speed and treated himself to a fast-food seafood dinner. But it does not strike unless it has a clear opportunity.

Cancer is an opportunistic disease in somewhat the same way. If conditions present an opportunity, any cell in the entire body can mutate. As we have already explained, mutations occur within the DNA. Malignant cells develop on a daily basis, but they are extinguished or reprogrammed back to being a normal cell by the body's natural defense system, if all is well.

Thus your body's natural defenses are your most important allies. In pristine condition, the human body is a strong fortress designed to fend off a frightening number of attacks daily. Any physician who tells you that keeping your body's defenses in tip-top shape is not the highest priority should be stripped of his license to practice.

Cancer is literally lying in wait, all the time, for any type of breakdown of the body's defense systems. When that opportunity comes, cell mutation will begin, and malignant cells will begin to reproduce at an uncontrollable, unstoppable rate. *Cancer is always a result of genetic abnormalities that are inherited or provoked by negative stressors.*

Should we fear the possibility of DNA fragmentation and cell mutation? No. We should dedicate ourselves to maintaining the normal, healthy functioning of our immune systems.

A Closer Look at the Immune System

The immune system is made up of organs and cells working as a team to protect the body from outside agents that could be harmful. Certain cells are able to distinguish between normal and abnormal cells. When an abnormal or foreign cell is detected, these cells seek them out and destroy them.

Many different types of cells make up the immune system. The specific cells that combat cancer are in the group called *lymphocytes*, which are one type of white blood cell that includes B cells, T cells, and natural killer (NK) cells.

T cells will directly attach to and attack cancerous cells. They are able to reproduce themselves through cloning right at the site of the abnormal cell. Also, they perform another important function. T cells sound the battle cry and call the NK cells into action. The NK cells are like little chemical factories that produce highly potent substances that attach themselves to and kill anything that is foreign to the body.

To complete the job, after the T and NK cells complete their destruction of cancer cells, macrophages and phagocytes absorb the dead cells and take them for elimination. This is why it is so important to make sure that the lymphatic system, which includes the liver, kidney, lungs, and bowels, is functioning properly.

Protecting White Blood Cells

What's the lesson here? Well, a properly functioning immune system provides the best way to prevent cancer on the front lines, because it's entirely natural. But it is also necessary to prevent a recurrence of cancer after other kinds of treatment have knocked it down or eliminated it. The problem with most conventional therapies, especially chemotherapy, is that they destroy the white blood cells.

For long-term remission of cancer, an adequate white blood cell count is indispensable. Fortunately, we have identified a natural substance called active hextose correlated compound (AHCC) that helps protect the white blood cell count, which we'll discuss at length in chapter nine.

Cancer Beater #5:
Address Your Immune System

We know that negative stressors generate damaging oxygen-free radicals that destabilize normal cells. Patients and physicians must put on their detective caps and try to at least identify the most obvious stressors that could be eliminated from the patient's lifestyle.

Most of the time, patients have to figure these things out themselves, because it takes a lot of time and concentrated thought. To help you do that, below is a list of internal and external stressors that are related to cancer. It is not comprehensive by any means. For example, more than thirty thousand carcinogens can be identified in the chemical industry alone. But consider the following as you look for ways to improve your lifestyle and surroundings.

Diet and nutritional factors (which represent 60 percent and 40 percent of all cancers in women and men, respectively)

- Fat intake
- High intake of animal protein
- Smoked foods
- Salt-cured foods
- Fried, broiled, or barbecued meat, chicken, or fish
- Pesticides found in food
- Food additives
- Alcohol
- High intake of caffeine

Smoking (which is the single major cause of cancer deaths, accounting for 30 percent of all deaths)

Environmental toxicity

- PCBs
- Garden pesticides
- Herbicides
- Contaminated soil, water, and air
- Asbestos
- Indoor pollution (fumes and vapors produced by cleaning products, paints, hobby supplies, and radon, among others)
- Chlorinated drinking water

Environmental radiation

- Electromagnetic fields
- Nuclear energy
- UV (solar) radiation
- Stress from psychological factors
- Depression

Genetics

Viruses

- Hepatitis B virus
- Herpes simplex 2
- CMV (Cytomegalovirus)

In Summary

Let's recap the concepts we have presented here:

1. The critical weakness of most treatments today is that they only attack the tumors. But tumors are just the symptoms of cancer. Granted, an effective program should try to reverse or halt the growth of tumors, but that will not be sufficient to avoid a relapse.

2. Immune function must be addressed as well, because a depressed immune system leaves the door wide open for cancer to come back, often with a vengeance. But this is still not enough. Immune dysfunction provides cancer the opportunity it needs to develop, but it is not its cause.

3. We should always try to detect what is stressing the body and its immune system. Potential stressors number in the

tens of thousands, so it may be impossible to identify the precise cause of a given patient's cancer. Other thousands of unknown causes must also be at work, which complicate things even further.

Considering the many thousands of cancer-causing agents out there, it is a miracle that everyone doesn't get cancer! And no wonder, indeed, that a cure-all "magic bullet" really doesn't exist. It is far more realistic to live our lives and take care of ourselves in ways that can either help beat/prevent cancer before it starts or slowly undo it once it has.

Throughout the rest of this book we will outline the ways you can minimize the negative affects of the stressors I have introduced very briefly above. Let's start with food.

Chapter 8

AVOID TOXIC FOODS AND HARMFUL SUBSTANCES

Cancer Beater #6

I N 1927, FOLLOWING THE COMPLAINTS OF A FORTY-TWO-YEAR-old woman, two doctors in Ontario, Canada, removed 2,533 objects, including 947 bent pins, from her stomach. In May 1985, doctors removed 212 objects from the stomach of a man in Cape Town, South Africa. The objects included 53 toothbrushes, 2 telescopic aerials, 2 razors, and 150 handles of disposable razors. Another man ground up and pulverized a bus over the period of several years and ate the entire vehicle![1]

The typical American diet is far more nourishing than the eccentric diets of these unfortunate individuals. Or is it? Think about your last trip to the local convenience store. You encountered a great deal of expensive food, but what nourishment did it offer?

You saw aisles and aisles of shiny packages of processed, fat-laden, sugary items of various shapes, sizes, and often amazingly unnatural colors. These "food" items included gooey pastries, orange-and-pink powdery chips, and bright blue drinks visually indistinguishable from commercial toilet cleaners in the next aisle.

Crossing over to the refrigerator section, perhaps you found frosty, premade sandwiches waiting for you, made with sticky, devitalized white bread that could wrap around your incisors like Super Glue, leaving you digging and scraping to clean your teeth so you could talk. Ugh!

On the other hand, maybe you found a shiny red apple! But it had been radiated to extend its shelf life, leaving barely enough vitamins and minerals to make crunching through the waxy pesticide coating worthwhile.

What has become of our food supply? Where is the vital nourishment that God intended for us when He said to Adam and Eve, "Behold, I have given you every plant yielding seed that is on the surface of all the earth, and every tree which has fruit yielding seed; it shall be food for you" (Gen. 1:29, NAS). Sadly, in terms of nutritional value, much of today's food bears greater resemblance to the eccentric diets of pins and screws we noted above than it does to the diet envisioned for us by our Creator.

We possess an enormous power over cancer—possibly enough to eradicate it completely—through prevention. Prevention is the most powerful tool we have with which to fight every disease and preserve life. The preservation of God's gift of health, I'm convinced, is a moral duty. But we cannot possibly fulfill that duty without knowing the level of actual nutrition the food we eat is actually giving to us.

Cancer Beater #6:
Avoid Toxic Foods

Until the end of the nineteenth century, most people lived off the land and depended on a very restricted, monotonous diet, yielded up by the crops of each season. Food was cultivated, gathered, cooked, and then eaten. There were few ways to store foods for any length of time.

But that all changed dramatically when the Industrial Revolution brought greater productivity and new methods for preserving food. Now the United States produces enough to feed the entire world, even while much of that world goes through famine.

Why? It is true that wars, droughts, floods, and other natural factors still ruin foodstuffs. But the ugly reality is that politics and economics are the real agricultural assassins. Food is now destroyed or stored to maintain its high market value, so that even when it is available, people around the globe cannot afford to buy what they need.

Meanwhile, in the world's industrialized countries, millions more overeat and waste their abundant food supply. Added to that is the sad reality that the food industry now gives us food that is increasingly electrified, fertilized, "pesticised," sterilized, refined, and processed. The devitalized foods we now eat, even in lands of plenty, give far less actual nourishment than the foods from earlier centuries.

Helping Mother Nature

We don't need to search very far to discover how increased productivity affects profits in the food business. Many producers increase productivity by manipulating nature with chemical fertilizers to shorten the harvest time. Others lay on the pesticides to diminish losses. Others increase their profits by distributing their product only when they can get the best prices instead of shortly after the harvest, when nutrients are at their highest levels.

But the best way industry giants have found to increase profit is to actually transform perishable food into imperishable food. In most cases, these methods severely damage the nutritional value of the food they produce; in other cases they erase virtually all of that value.

Foods grown today are processed with three objectives in view: to be tasty, precooked, and indestructible. Many of these imperishable foods can stay on your shelf or in your refrigerator for months and still be edible. Such "high-profit" foods are the backbone of the food industry, dressed up in shiny, appealing packages. But they offer little more nutritional value than the pretty wrappings they come in.

Hunger in the affluent societies of the world is tastefully, conveniently, and artificially answered by the food industry. The fastest-growing companies within the food industry are fast-food (processed, precooked) corporations. Throughout the world fast-food restaurants are continually opening. And every year the food industry spends additional millions to increase demand for its products.

Meanwhile, our bodies cry out for nutritious food to meet the challenges of a modern existence, including the threat of cancer and a host of other degenerative diseases. Contrary to popular belief, eating should not be just a recreational activity. We should eat with great care, focusing our full attention on making sure we get the nutrients we need for good health.

And all the while, the fast foods creatively produced to save us minutes in our days steal years from our lives.

Nutrients Out; Poisons In!

Today, not only is the land overused and depleted, but also the most frequently used fertilizers destroy iron, vitamin C, folic acid, minerals, lysine, amino acids, and many other nutrients. Pesticides contaminate the soil and take a long time to disappear. For example, a chemical called chlordane was once used indiscriminately in pesticides by commercial growers. Even though it has been virtually banned since 1988, chlordane has a half-life of twenty years. This means that after twenty years it will still be half as strong as it was when it was applied to the soil.

Remember that all plants absorb the substances found in the earth in which they grow. While authorities have finally prohibited many pesticides proven to be strong carcinogens, the weak carcinogenic pesticides are still considered safe (but only to a scientist paid by the pesticide industry). In the laboratories they are tested individually. But in real life they are never used alone. These chemicals are combined with others, which dramatically increases their cancer-causing effects.

Today, pesticides contaminate more than 94 percent of the foods we eat. Without a doubt, continuous exposure to them can cause cancer and other degenerative diseases. In 1968, a research group found that patients who died from liver cancer, brain cancer, multiple sclerosis, and other degenerative diseases had significantly higher traces of pesticides in their brains and fatty tissue than those who had died from other diseases.[2]

Some of the pesticides considered less toxic can still cause depression, migraines, hyperactivity, and more. Pesticides are easily absorbed and hard to eliminate; they remain in our bodies with dire effects because of their chemical affinity to estrogen (as we will discuss later).

"Incorruptible" Produce

A couple of years ago, a family friend purchased their traditional pumpkin for the harvest season. After Thanksgiving, they placed it in their garage where it sat, and sat—and sat! It seemed it would never spoil. For months they kept checking it, wondering how much longer the "super" pumpkin would last. It became a little game.

Finally, several months later they threw it into the trash, more out of boredom than because it had yielded to the corruption of all living things. It might still be sitting there today. Indeed, it could well be sitting at the dump even yet, looking just as it did then. My friend concluded that the tennis racket leaning on the wall next to the pumpkin would have decayed sooner.

What Makes Bacteria Thrive?

To realize the negative impact of such produce on our bodies, we need to understand what makes food rot and biodegrade. The answer is nothing more or less than bacterial invasion—when bacteria start eating food, the food rots. In other words, bacteria feed on the same nutrients our bodies need to survive. If there are no nutrients in the food, or if it contains poisons, bacteria stay away, and the food does not rot.

Do you get the picture? Even bacteria won't "eat" devitalized or poisoned food. Should you? Conversely, if bacteria beat you to the food, at least you know it was free of poisons and rich in nutrients; it was not only edible, but it was also nutritious.

My friends' immortal pumpkin had undoubtedly been irradiated, which is another way that the food industry manipulates the food we eat and causes bacteria to leave it alone. The food industry has learned to use radiation to sanitize produce, which increases profits by prolonging shelf life. However, the radioisotopes they use do more than just destroy nutrients. Their particles easily enter into our living cells, where they increase the risk of cell mutation and cancer.

What Bugs Know About Wheat

In the same way that bacteria know what kinds of food they need to eat, insects seem to know something about the same subject.

For many generations, wheat was the staff of life for cultures around the world. It supplied a rich, highly accessible source of protein, amino acids, complex carbohydrates, and fiber.

Today, about 678 million metric tons of wheat are harvested worldwide each year, but our bodies no longer benefit in the same ways from this wonderful natural product. Wheat has been handed a death sentence by the food processors—it has been completely devitalized, stripped of its nutrients and its ability to nourish our bodies.

Just think—you no longer need to worry about how long it's been sitting on your pantry shelf! Whether it's been there for two weeks or two years, you won't find bugs in your flour or your bread. In this respect, bugs may be smarter than we are. They refuse to eat what doesn't nourish them.

The flour you eat is as dead as the ground-up bus eaten by the man we mentioned earlier. When wheat is refined, it loses:

- 80 percent of its vitamin B_1 (thiamin)
- 80 percent of its vitamin B_2 (riboflavin)
- 80 percent of its vitamin B_3 (niacin) and vitamin B_6
- 98 percent of its vitamin E
- 90 percent of its minerals and micronutrients
- 80 percent of its biotin
- 76 percent of its vitamin K

- 75 percent of its folic acid

- 50 percent of its linoleic acid

- 99 percent of its fiber

- 100 percent of about twenty-seven other nutrients

The only "benefit" is that the refining process increases wheat's caloric value by 7 percent! Obviously, appearance is everything.

Only for Appearance's Sake

Another consideration of the food industry is that the average consumer demands produce that "looks good." To protect them from dents, scrapes, and bruises, fruits and vegetables are specially boxed or piled. Never mind that when they are picked and left outside more than two or three hours, their nutritional value is reduced by 40 to 50 percent.

Potatoes lose up to 78 percent of their vitamin C within a week after they are harvested. Spinach greens, asparagus, broccoli, and peas lose 50 percent of their vitamins before they ever get to market. Packaging and transporting produce compromises its nutritional value even more. And produce sitting in storage loses additional nutrients.

To increase shelf life and appearance, farmers harvest their fruits and vegetables long before they are mature. That might seem innocent enough, for we have gradually lowered our expectations regarding flavor. But fruits and vegetables absorb most of their vitamins and minerals when they are almost ripe. The next time you pick up a bunch of bright green bananas, think about this: they will never fill up with the vitamins and minerals they would have acquired ripening in the sun rather than sitting on supermarket shelves or your kitchen counter!

So once again nutrition takes a back seat—this time to appearance. Unfortunately, appearance may be just about all this deficient produce gives you.

The Wonders of Processed Foods

Processed foods are even more profitable than manipulated produce, simply because they last longer. The twin goals of availability and convenience move the industry to provide imperishable, user-friendly foods in cans, cartons, or frozen bags. But in every step of the process, vital nutrients are sacrificed.

Juices and milk are often packaged in containers lined with wax, a known cancer-causing substance. Plastic containers aren't much better since they are made from petrochemicals (polymers with toxic stabilizers and color tinctures such as acrylic acid), tuolene, Styrofoam, and vinyl chloride. These carcinogens abound in disposable plates, bowls, and cups as well.

Most frozen vegetables lose 25 percent of vitamins A, B_1, B_2, C, and niacin, among others, during the freezing process. Broccoli, cauliflower, peas, and spinach lose up to 50 percent of theirs.

Canned foods lose more than 50 percent of all nutrients during the canning process. In addition, the nitrites that are added to kill botulism, when heated with the food, are converted into nitrosamines, another potent cancer-causing substance.

By the time these "new tech" foods get to our mouths, they have already been sprayed with acidifiers, alkalinizers, antifoaming agents, artificial colors, artificial flavors, sweeteners, deodorants, fillers, disinfectants, emulsifiers, extenders, hydrogenators, moisturizers, and plenty more. As a final insult, they are laced with *synthetic* vitamins to replace chemically what has been lost!

No wonder bacteria will not touch the stuff. Modern profit-generating foods are so "well made" that they are practically indestructible!

Eating Preservatives

Unobstructed by authorities, backed by investors, encouraged by profits, and waved on by our ignorance, food producers have raced down the path of chemical chaos, adding ever-increasing amounts of preservatives to our foods. In the 1960s, Americans consumed about three pounds per person per year of these noxious chemicals. In the 1970s, that number rose to about six pounds, and since then we have crossed the ten-pound line.[3]

Curiously, health officials are not alarmed by the increase in morbidity and mortality caused by fast and convenient *un*-foods. Morticians, however, are astonished to find corpses that should have converted to ashes long ago, still as fresh as a newly picked lettuce! They report that the average cadaver takes twice as long to decompose today as it did thirty years ago. What a phenomenon! Food preservatives that accelerate our trip to the grave give us the macabre advantage of keeping us presentable longer in our tombs! If only the pharaohs knew.

Raising the Sacred Cow

Even before cowboys began to sit around campfires at night singing "Home on the Range" to their steers, Americans already loved meat. The demand for beef and other meats has steadily increased through the years. As a result, the food industry has developed scientific methods to increase the production of red and white meats.

In 1940 it took more than four pounds of feed to produce one pound of meat. In the 1980s it took only two pounds.[4] Sixty years ago, a cow produced two thousand pounds of milk per year. Today, milk producers get fifty thousand pounds of milk per year per cow.[5]

How have such marvelous increases in production been achieved? The modern livestock industry has created super chickens and monster cows through chemically enhanced feeds, genetic engineering, drugs, and hormones.

Consumers now have access to the information about most of what they are ingesting, thanks to recent FDA labeling regulations. But despite strong complaints, livestock producers have had preferential treatment and are not required to list the additives and ingredients in their products. This encourages consumers to assume that meat is meat and milk is, well, milk. Right?

Actually, the FDA allows the administration of up to eighty-two drugs to cows during the production of dairy products.[6] Among these drugs, the *bovine growth hormone* and *estrogen* are the most abused. And of these, the most harmful to humans is the female hormone estrogen.

Scientific research suggests that the effects of bovine growth hormone and estrogen together on the body can cause arthritis, obesity, glucose intolerance, diabetes, and heart disease. They may also be responsible for other less serious but annoying maladies, including headaches, fatigue, vision impairment, dizziness, menstrual problems, and loss of sexual drive.[7]

Let me hasten to add that meat and milk are not bad for you; otherwise, God would not have recommended them to us. What has become a menace to our health is their profitable adulteration by the food industry. Fortunately, more and more organically produced meat and milk are being made available.

Estrogen Contamination

The harmful effects I listed above, caused by estrogen and estrogen-like substances, account for much of the modern litany of "dis-ease." Just about all our foods contain pesticides. Most of these pesticides have a chemical structure very closely related to that of estrogen—close enough to fool our bodies. When we eat pesticide-tainted foods, they provoke a weak estrogenic effect on our systems.

For example, the plastics that wrap and keep our foods fresh also produce mild effects similar to what estrogen would produce in our bodies. Since those effects are weak, we consider such products safe. But when so many of the materials and foods around us have been tainted, the compounded effect becomes significantly stronger. The consequences of the combined estrogenic effect of all of these products can be powerful.

A good example would be the livestock contamination that occurred on a Michigan farm. Here the livestock feed was contaminated with the pesticide polychlorinated biphenyl (PCB), which is considered a "weak" estrogen imitator. However, pregnant women and mothers who consumed the meat of these animals and then breast-fed their children were horrified to find that their male children developed genital deformities and very small penises.[8]

In Taiwan, Chinese scientists have under observation 118 male children of mothers who were contaminated with PCB in an accidental spill in 1989. These boys suffer from the same painful complications as the boys from the Michigan farm contamination.[9]

In lakes with high concentrations of DDT and DDE—pesticides that also have estrogenic effects—the fauna have been severely degenerated. Alligators of Lake Apopka in Florida have lost virility because of low testosterone and sperm count; their male organs are 25 percent smaller than the norm. The Great Lakes are gravely polluted with PCB and DDT; the result is that many fish and seagulls that get their food there have developed grotesque hormonal dysfunctions that make them hermaphrodites, according to Theo Colburn of the World Wildlife Fund.[10]

Niels Skakkebaek, a Danish endocrinologist and probably the foremost authority on the subject of estrogen, reported in 1991 that because of exaggerated exposure to estrogen and estrogen-like substances, men presently have only 50 percent of the normal sperm count. They also are experiencing a significant reduction in the size of their reproductive organs, and the incidence of testicular cancer has tripled.[11]

These chemicals have mercilessly maimed our society. Synthetic estrogens and the chemical agents that mimic estrogen represent a very real threat to our health. They do not break down easily, and our bodies cannot neutralize them. They end up tainting our entire food chain and remain active for many years.

But of course, the damage is not limited to men. Long Island, New York, has one of the highest incidences of breast cancer in the United States. Experts believe this is due to the vast quantity of pesticides used on the farming soils before they were converted to urban communities. Today, these pesticides are still abundant in the local tap water.

Mary Wolf, MD, a professor at Mt. Sinai School of Medicine in New York, reported that breast tumor biopsies of women from Long Island showed unusually high concentrations of DDT and DDE. And the incidence of cancer was four times higher than in biopsies where the pesticides were absent or in low concentrations.[12] Research overwhelmingly suggests that estrogen increases the incidence of many female ailments, including cancer of the breast, uterus, and ovaries.

Sadly, cancer is only one of the disorders that an excess of artificially added estrogens has brought upon women. Menstrual, fertility, ovarian, and uterine problems can be listed as well. German scientists have also discovered high blood concentrations of PCB in women suffering with endometriosis, an inflammatory pelvic disease that causes severe pain and sterility. Before pesticides arrived on the scene, endometriosis was virtually unheard of. In 1920, only twenty-one cases were reported worldwide. Today, upwards of five million women battle this painful problem in the United States alone.

The Nightmare of Nitrates

Purchasing gray or brown meat from your favorite grocer would probably not be very appealing. If you are like most shoppers, you look for bright red meat as an indicator of freshness. However, you may already be aware that the red color doesn't really indicate freshness anymore. Today's meat is packed with nitrates to make it look fresher as it sits on the shelf.

Nitrates, a pillar of the meat industry, become serious cancer-causing agents when they are heated. Nitrates are also widely used in the preparation of lunch meats, hot dogs, and bacon. It's been shown that children who eat twelve or more hot dogs a month are 9.5 times as likely to get leukemia.[13] When pregnant mothers eat hot dogs during pregnancy, the incidence of brain cancer in their children increases dramatically as well.[14]

One of the only truly natural things left in our meat is the fat—and there's plenty of that. Nearly 60 percent of meat and dairy products, including milk, eggs, cheese, and processed meats, is now fat. The fatty meats and dairy products we consume tend to trap the toxic chemicals and antibiotics, dramatically increasing our risk of obesity, hypertension, cardiovascular diseases, hyperthyroidism, candidiasis, and cancer. Of the 143 chemical substances found in commercial meats, 42 are cancer causing or carcinogenic, and 20 more can cause birth defects.[15]

Vegetable Oils Unmasked

Animal fats have been considered so harmful that, many years ago, health experts began to recommend vegetable oils instead, obtained from grains, seeds, and nuts. For centuries vegetable oils have been used around the world for nutritional, medicinal, and religious purposes. Through simple compression of the plants or grains you can obtain oils of excellent quality.

However, because they also contain an enormous amount of nutrients, these natural vegetable oils tend to spoil very quickly, and they are also very appealing to bacteria. Therefore, to increase the shelf life of vegetable oil, experts developed a process called mechanical extraction. In this process pressure mills crush the seeds and then heat the mash to 240 degrees. Afterward, the unrefined oil is pressed at more than twenty tons of pressure per square inch. This removes all the elements that can spoil. Unfortunately, all the nutritional value is also lost. Today's vegetable oils have no more nutritional value than the motor oil in your car.

To create a less-expensive process for extracting oil from grains, scientists next developed a chemical extraction method. Seeds are heated to 160 degrees and then allowed to rest in gasoline, hexane, ethylene, carbon disulfide, tetrachloride, or methyl chloride. Afterward, the solvent is evaporated, though a very minute portion remains mixed with the oil. Then the carotene is removed through a chlorination process, yielding crystal-clear oil.

Although this process is able to extend the shelf life almost indefinitely, it also destroys any nutritional value. Even worse, it makes the fatty acids toxic. Margarine and vegetable shortening are hydrogenated and made solid by high pressure and heating the oil to 380 degrees. Our bodies cannot metabolize these substances, which also hinder them from using other oils we need.

Fake Fats

In January 1996, the Food and Drug Administration gave Proctor and Gamble permission to sell snack foods, such as chips, fried in Olean (the trademark name for olestra, which is a fake fat). Olean is a proven anti-nutrient. In other words, not only does it not give anything nutritious to your body, but also it actually robs nutrition *from* the body.

Olean is designed to look and taste like fat, but unlike fat, it cannot be absorbed into the body from the intestinal tract. It runs freely through your gastrointestinal tract, unabsorbed, and is passed out in the feces. It may cause anal leakage, and as fat passes through the intestines unabsorbed, fat-soluble nutrients attach to it and are carried out also. Among these fat-soluble nutrients that are lost are beta-carotene, a cancer fighter, and other carotenoids. Studies reveal that upwards of 40 percent of carotenoids may be reduced by eating Olean.[16]

Fake diet foods such as Olean do not actually reduce obesity. In fact, they have been linked to weight gain.

A Nutrient Death Sentence

Many of the foods we eat have long since been handed a nutritional death sentence by the food processing industry. Refined sugar, refined flour, and processed oils make up the core of this industry. They cost almost nothing to produce, they last forever on the shelf, and they are the primary ingredients in all processed foods.

Sugar was the first food to receive the deathblow. About two hundred years ago, profiteers discovered they could "purify" sugar of any elements that might cause it to decompose without taking away its sweetness. They called the process "refining." Refining sugar strips it entirely of its nutritional value, creating naked calories. Refined sugar is composed of 96 percent sucrose, 3 percent waste, 1 percent water, and 0 percent nutrition.

Another example of "naked calories" is corn syrup. Corn syrup is also an anti-nutrient. It has zero nutritional value, and it robs the body of nutrients such as thiamin, riboflavin, and niacin.

Since its arrival in 1751, refined sugar has been the most consumed food stock worldwide. We start taking in refined sugar almost from birth. Until recently it was not even unusual for nurses to give sugar water to newborns who were waiting for their mothers to recuperate from childbirth!

Sugars enter your body and are almost instantly rushed to your brain and heart, giving these organs an immediate feeling of energy and well-being. Sugar also robs the body of calcium, thereby promoting tooth decay. And sugar creates a dependency as strong as any other addictive drug. If you stop eating sugar completely, you are likely to experience withdrawal symptoms.

The typical high-sugar American diet comes with an enormous price tag of neurosis, hypoglycemia, diabetes mellitus, cancer of the biliary tract, colorectal cancer, arthritis, arteriosclerosis, coronary insufficiency, and more. Yet the average American consumes 170 pounds of sugar annually.[17] In other words, most people eat more than their entire body weight in sugar in one year!

You may think those estimates don't include you because you don't eat a lot of candy. The fact is that most of that sugar intake—a whopping 66 percent—comes camouflaged in processed un-foods. Even with increased public awareness, the average individual continues to derive 25 percent of all his or her calories from sugar.

You might think that it would not be difficult to eat less than 30 pounds of sugar a year—one-fourth of the entire body weight of a small- to medium-sized woman. Eating this moderate amount of sugar would ensure you of less illness and a strong tendency to live longer. For example, the Seventh-Day Adventists eat a vegetarian diet and avoid preservatives and refined foods. Surely it is no coincidence that they live an average of twelve years longer than the rest of the population.

The Death of Fiber

The most severe death sentence handed to our food supply from the food industry was the death of fiber. Fiber never stood a chance—it has been virtually wiped out.

Living cancer free and maintaining a general state of good health depends on our capacity to adequately nourish ourselves and eliminate waste efficiently. Fiber has the life-saving task of helping our bodies eliminate waste. Without proper elimination, dangerous and poisonous toxins remain inside our bodies, becoming increasingly rancid. If we cannot expel them quickly, our bodies are left with little choice but to reabsorb the poisons that our systems tried to reject. This toxic state, as we have already seen, is the seedbed of cancer.

The result of our fiber-poor diet is a chronically constipated society. This condition has perpetuated itself so strongly that even in medical schools they teach us that moving our bowels between once a day and once every three days is normal.

Researchers like H. S. Goldsmith and E. L. Wynder reported that people in our modern Western culture produce small amounts of feces every twenty-four to forty-eight hours. These stools are hard, segmented, and frequently painful and difficult to excrete.

This compares to people who eat primitive diets, fiber-rich in raw fruits and vegetables, who eliminate three times as much waste with soft and voluminous feces that are easy to excrete. And while Westerners finally defecate the remains of food they ate two days earlier, groups like the Hunza people report a maximum intestinal transit time of ten hours.

Kian Liu and E. L. Wynder discovered that for every 100,000 inhabitants in the United States, 109 die of colon cancer, but only 4 of every 100,000 in Uganda die of the same thing.[18] This is the quantitative difference between the modern, high-tech diet and a fiber-rich diet. Although their eating habits are very different, virtually all Ugandans live a long time and are seldom ill. The secret? They have very high-fiber diets that prevent constipation and efficiently detoxify their bodies from dangerous, cancer-causing poisons.

English experts like J. Yudkin from London, in 1972 and later in 1974, and T. L. Cleave from Bristol reported a high incidence of cancer in peoples from the modern Western world because of diets rich in fats and refined foods, resulting in constipation. Later T. D. Wilkins and A. S. Hackman published similar findings with respect to Americans.[19] Their feces contained elevated quantities of nitrogen, fat, cholesterol, biliary acids, and a high concentration of carcinogenic metabolites, which are chemical wastes produced as our body metabolizes the adulterated food.

Dr. Adlercreutz, in his article "Diet, Mammary Cancer and Metabolism of the Sex Hormone," underlines the fact that Western women enjoy unrestrained consumption of animal proteins and fats, along with refined carbohydrates. This low-fiber diet increases their risk of colon cancer and also substantially increases the production of estrogens. This excessive endogenous estrogen—which normally should be eliminated through the stool—is trapped in the colon by constipation and is easily reabsorbed into the bloodstream.

In contrast, Asian women who eat high-fiber, unprocessed foods avoid this deadly cycle. Their hormones tend to be much more stable because of their superior diet and good detoxification. It is now commonly accepted that high-fiber diets increase expectancy for good health.

Meanwhile, though we have pointed the finger at harmful estrogen and estrogenic chemicals, we must note that not all estrogens are harmful. Vegetables such as soybeans, broccoli, and pomegranates offer us phytohormones or phytoestrogens, which protect us from carcinogenic mutations. Typically, diets that contain good amounts of these and other phytoestrogen-rich foods help to fight against disease. Chinese and Japanese women eat foods rich in good estrogen, such as tofu, soy, and miso. They seldom develop cancer, and curiously, they rarely suffer osteoporosis or any of the diseases related to low estrogen production after menopause.

Mental Havoc

Our generation has been fed on processed, devitalized, dead foods. As a result, we have become one of the most overfed and undernourished cultures on Earth. Our diet has exposed us to cancer and other degenerative diseases that might otherwise have been prevented.

Children are especially affected by our poor diet in dramatic ways. Their bodies need plenty of rich, wholesome food that they are not getting. Instead, they are growing up in today's fast-food, junk-food world. Teeth, cells, bones, muscles, and vital tissue are being built from materials that are worse than inferior. In many respects they are deadly, as we have discussed.

The consequences of our lack of proper nutrition don't stop with increased threats of physical disease. Eating dead, toxic food has affected our intellectual abilities as well. A serious increase in behavioral problems in children and adolescents can be directly attributed to poor nutrition.

Hyper-aggression in our youth is linked to eating refined sugars found in sweets and sodas.[20] Modern jails are showcases for this behavioral problem. In one of them, a dietary experiment was carried out in which fruit, fresh vegetables, and water were substituted for sweets, cookies, and sodas. Aggressiveness and other behavior problems among the prisoners were reduced remarkably in just a couple of weeks![21]

It's hard not to think of Daniel and the healthful results he and his friends achieved by turning down the rich foods of King Nebuchadnezzar in the Old Testament! But again, here in more modern times, this simple, inexpensive "jailhouse" experiment clearly demonstrates the relationship between behavioral problems and diet.

Vitamin and mineral deficiencies affect the biochemical balance that controls the neurotransmitters in the brain. According to researchers from Massachusetts Institute of Technology, this crucial alteration leads to learning and behavioral dysfunction.[22] This is by no means a new discovery. In 1790 (not 1970), at the Tuke's Clinic in York, England, complete wards of patients diagnosed with dementia were emptied when a regimen of nutritious foods was implemented.[23]

In Summary

In addition to dealing with the nutritional deficiency issues introduced by the modern diet, we must also address the toxicity problem it introduces into the body. If the body does not get rid of built-up toxins, it will not be able to heal as it should. That's why avoiding toxic foods is cancer beater #6.

Toxins that are currently being put into the bodies of the majority of people in the Western world are the two cancer beaters we've addressed in this chapter. First, avoid *toxic* foods, meaning:

- Foods void of nutrition

- Foods that include additives, preservatives, and artificial ingredients that harm the body

- Foods that sludge the digestive tract, depress the immune system, excite the nervous system, and in general remove the possibility of health

In other words, the standard diet most people consume, which is a diet high in:

- Animal products—meat and dairy

- White flour products—pasta, breads, and cakes

- Refined white sugar products—candy bars, sodas, and other sweets

- Refined salt

In addition, through the consumption of legal drugs such as caffeine, nicotine, alcohol, artificial sweeteners, and prescription drugs, even as the body tries to get healthy we continue adding to its burden.

The China Project[24] showed a strong correlation between the incidence of cancer and the amount of animal foods consumed. According to the research:

> Carcinogenesis—the development of cancer—is turned on by animal protein and turned off by plant protein, even if cancer has already been initiated. It appears that once the body has all the protein it needs—about 8 percent to 10 percent of the entire diet—then excess protein begins to feed precancerous lesions and tumors.[25]

When we eliminate these toxic substances (including the animal foods with their excess protein) and replace them with nutritious foods and fresh juices, we give the body what it needs to heal itself, regardless of the diagnosed disease.

Remember, *a diagnosis is just a name given to a collection of symptoms.* In turn, the symptoms are indicators from the body that it is facing toxicity and/or deficiency, which the immune system has not been able to heal. Our responsibility is to build up the body and the immune system and to furnish it with whatever it needs to rid itself of not only the symptoms but the underlying causes as well.

In addition to toxins put into our bodies through food, we need to also be aware of the environmental toxins in our air and water, pesticides on our foods, and other external sources to which we are exposed. It is essential to minimize these toxins as much as possible to help facilitate healing.

Current medical treatment utilizes toxic substances to treat cancer, but I don't believe we should submit a patient's body to aggressive surgeries, radiation, and chemotherapy when their immune systems are already suppressed from cancer. When these invasive techniques are used, the body must divert valuable energy away from dealing with the cancer to deal with what it sees as a threat to basic survival—the treatment.

Also, although it puts a great deal of focus on the nutritional component, the Hallelujah diet (see the next chapter) introduces more than just a change in the foods we eat. It is a total lifestyle change involving every aspect of life—spiritual, emotional, and physical. It is vital to include sunshine; fresh air; pure water; adequate rest (the body does most of its healing when we sleep); exercise (cancer cells cannot survive in an oxygenated environment); a positive mental outlook; dealing with issues of anger, bitterness, and hostility; and, most important, a trusting, loving relationship with God.

There is not one thing that causes cancer and other chronic diseases—they generally result from a combination of internal toxins, external toxins, malnutrition, stressful living, and many other contributors. In the same way, nutrition alone cannot overcome cancer, and neither can exercise, pure water, or any other single change. By addressing *all areas* we provide the best environment for healing to take place, just as God intended back in the Garden of Eden. And that is where healing begins—with God, and through obedience to the natural laws He gave us.

Chapter 9

EAT FOODS THAT CAN HEAL YOU

Cancer Beaters #7–9

SITTING IN FRONT OF MY COMPUTER, SURROUNDED BY SCORES OF scientific papers, health books, and a head full of bright ideas (at least I think they're bright!), I (Francisco Contreras) find it quite easy to chastise you and make recommendations for your healthy lifestyle. However, I recognize that walking the aisles of modern food stores confronts us all with the food industry's single most powerful and tempting allure: convenience!

For every real food item your grocer sells, he offers hundreds of un-food choices, most of which are tastier and more conveniently packaged.

I ask myself, "What would bacteria do if they entered one of our modern supermarkets?" Then I answer my own question: they would run for their lives unless the food store had an organically grown food section. Fortunately, in the United States this inconvenient and more expensive organic section is becoming more and more popular. Though paying the price and caring for these real foods does require some sacrifice, we still seem to be seeing constantly increasing demand for real foods, as more people make the right choices and enjoy the benefits they bring.

However, radical change is not always necessary and definitely should not be the first thing you try in order to escape from the typical "dead food" American diet. Start by eliminating a few toxic foods and adding a few living foods. This alone will aid your body's built-in healing processes immensely.

Meanwhile, let me present my favorite diet, which is a great way of eating to help prevent all kinds of disease. In the next chapter I will provide a deeper look into the world of super-foods, and I will present a *therapeutic* diet that is much stricter and possibly can reverse cancer, heart disease, and almost every other kind of chronic ailment.

Cancer Beater #7:
The Mediterranean Diet

The "French paradox," as it is known in scientific circles, is the enigma that the life expectancy of the French people, compared to Americans, is longer. Considering that the French eat more fat and consume more red wine than Americans, many scientists cannot understand why they experience fewer heart attacks and a lower incidence of cancer, spend one-third the money on health care as Americans, and yet enjoy a longer life span.

Well, the technocrats cannot take credit for this paradox, because the longevity of the French is not a result of medical and technological advances. It is a direct result of ancient cultural dietary habits.

Of course, not all the peoples of the Mediterranean countries eat exactly the same diet. But their rates of coronary heart disease and cancer are significantly lower than they are for people in America, with the lowest death rates and longer life expectancy among these Mediterranean cultures occurring in Greece. Though the typical Greek diet is similar to that of other Mediterranean peoples, it differs in the amount of total fat and olive oil they consume, the types of meat they eat, their wine intake, their milk-versus-cheese ratio, and their intake of fruits and vegetables. Here are the common denominators of the Mediterranean diet:

- High monounsaturated/saturated fat ratio (olive oil)

- Moderate alcohol consumption (red wine during meals)

- High consumption of legumes
- High consumption of whole grains
- High consumption of fruits
- High consumption of vegetables
- Low consumption of meat and meat products
- Moderate consumption of milk and dairy products

Extensive studies of traditional diets indicate that a typical Greek person's diet includes a high intake of fruits, vegetables (particularly wild plants), nuts, and cereals (mostly in the form of sourdough bread rather than pasta); more olive oil and olives; less milk but more cheese; more fish; less meat; and moderate amounts of wine, but more than in other Mediterranean countries.[1]

"Natural" supplements

The foods that the people of Mediterranean cultures consume are, in general, not only pesticide and chemically free, but they are also loaded with natural cancer-fighting and heart-friendly agents. These include selenium, glutathione, a balanced ratio of omega-6 to omega-3 essential fatty acids, high amounts of fiber, and antioxidants such as vitamins E and C, which have been shown to be associated with a lower risk of cancer, including cancer of the breast.

A little wine, please

Resveratrol (found in grapes and wine and polyphenols from olive oil) is a promising anticancer agent for both hormone-dependent and hormone-independent breast cancers, and it may mitigate the growth stimulatory effect of linoleic acid in the Western-style diet.[2]

Phytochemicals found in grapes and wine, like resveratrol, have also been reported to bring about a variety of anti-inflammatory, anti-platelet, and anticarcinogenic effects.[3]

A nutty snack

Instead of snacking on high-caloric, fat-laden, chemical-rich, processed junk food, Mediterranean people quiet their between-meal appetites by eating nuts. This is very smart, because studies have reported that almond consumption may reduce colon cancer risk. Western dieticians, ignorant of the health benefits of nuts, have scared us away from eating them because of their high fat and caloric content. Nonetheless, almonds and other nuts appear to confer important health benefits.[4]

Bring on the tomato sauce

Tomato sauce (not ketchup), one of the main ingredients of the Mediterranean diet and the primary source of bioavailable lycopene, a carotenoid from tomatoes, is associated with an even greater reduction in prostate cancer risk, especially for the more aggressive and life-threatening extraprostatic cancers. Harvard Medical School researchers reported in the *Journal of the National Cancer Institute* that lycopene intake was associated with reduced risk of prostate cancer.[5]

Cancer prevention diet

Dr. Jang, from the department of surgical oncology at the University of Illinois at Chicago, says that the Mediterranean diet has the potential to prevent cancer at each of the three major stages of its development.[6]

1. Anti-initiation activity was indicated by its antioxidant and antimutagenic effects, inhibition of the hydroperoxidase function of cyclooxygenase (COX), and induction of phase II drug-metabolizing enzymes.

2. Antipromotion activity was indicated by anti-inflammatory effects, inhibition of production of arachidonic acid metabolites catalyzed by either COX-1 or COX-2, and chemical carcinogen-induced neoplastic transformation of mouse embryo fibroblasts.

3. Antiprogression activity was demonstrated by its ability to induce human promyelocytic leukemia (HL-60) cell differentiation.

It seems to me that the results of this research should serve as a strong incentive to the scientific community to test the effects of specific dietary patterns in the prevention and management of patients with cancer. Unfortunately, instead of learning from these tangible proofs, we continue to search for the elusive magic bullet. To say the least, the politics and economics of the cancer industry seem to cloud the minds of even our best-intentioned scientists.

You may wonder if I recommend any other type of diet. Actually, any diet high in vegetable- and fruit-derived fiber and low in animal fat and protein would be good. Thus, diets such as the macrobiotic diet and the vegan diet are definitely worth considering. The Gerson therapy, a food-based therapy, has also brought relief to thousands of cancer patients. These are all excellent for prevention.

Cancer Beater #8: The Hallelujah Diet

Over the years I have been impressed by the countless testimonies of people who reversed their cancer through adhering to the amazingly effective Hallelujah diet. I will warn you that if you are used to steak and potatoes, hamburgers, french fries, and soda, when you switch to the raw vegetables and fruits that make up the Hallelujah diet, you will feel challenged at first. But your life is worth it![7]

Dr. George Malkmus designed the Hallelujah diet based on the premise that, as our Creator, God gave us guidelines for every aspect of our lives, including how to live healthy and avoid disease. He created our bodies to live forever, placing within us an innate capability for self-healing.

Thus the purpose of the Hallelujah diet is twofold: first, to rectify the nutrient deficiency—malnutrition; and second, to eliminate the toxicity that occurs in our bodies.

By doing these two things, the Hallelujah diet helps bring our bodies back into balance, or *homeostasis*, as God's design intended. Then all the built-in healing processes can occur automatically. When the immune system functions optimally, cancer does not develop.

On the other hand, when cancer has already developed because of an impaired immune system, it may be possible to reverse such cancer development as we rebuild the system through optimal nutrition and lifestyle changes.

To address nutrient deficiency, the Hallelujah diet stresses the importance of consuming foods in their natural state—raw and preferably organically grown. The body then benefits from the enzymes, vitamins, minerals, proteins, and other nutrients present in living foods.

For example, phytochemicals in their natural state, such as lycopene in tomatoes and peppers, have been shown to be potent cancer inhibitors. Cruciferous vegetables such as broccoli and cauliflower are high in isothiocyanates, which activate enzymes present in all cells that detoxify carcinogens.[8]

We believe that the quality of the food we provide is so important that at Oasis of Hope our medical director has taken the time to work with farm owners nearby to ensure that the food they supply us is grown organically, without pesticides, and is delivered directly from the farm to the hospital a number of times per week.

Dr. Joel Fuhrman, in his book *Eat to Live*, explains how food rich in the nutrition our bodies need enables them to work toward health restoration.

> When we consume a sufficient variety and quantity of phytochemical substances we afford ourselves the ability to repair DNA damage, detoxify cancer-causing agents, and resist disease in general.[9]

In essence, through eating a diet high in living foods, we provide our bodies with everything that they need to properly nourish their cells, enabling them to begin rebuilding and repairing damaged cells, tissues, and ultimately their organs as well.

Cancer Beater #9:
Eat Other Cancer-Fighting, Natural Foods

Beyond all the above, the study of functional whole foods and natural, disease-fighting substances is just beginning. Despite what the food industry has wrought, with respect to natural, organically grown foods that can still help you fight against cancer, the modern medical community has barely opened the door of nature's medicine chest. I encourage you to get online and learn as much as you can about these things and put them to work for your health. Eating can be therapeutic and enjoyable if you eat the right things.

Tomatoes

To begin with, the tomato is one of the richest sources of a powerful antioxidant we have already mentioned called lycopene. Antioxidants are substances that scavenge free radicals. Remember, free radicals can damage cells and the gene expression process. Therefore tomatoes are rich in the stuff that may prevent cancer from beginning.

Several epidemiological studies show that the regular intake of tomatoes and tomato products is associated with a lower risk of several cancers. One case-control study of an elderly population linked the consistent intake of tomato lycopene to protective effects against digestive tract cancers and a 50 percent reduction in death from cancer.[10]

Dr. Edward Giovannucci reviewed seventy-two epidemiological studies.[11] These included ecological, case-control, dietary, and blood-specimen-based investigations. All the studies examined the effect of tomato lycopene on cancer. In the majority, the researchers found an inverse association between tomato intake and the risk of several types of cancer.

In other words, the more tomatoes a person ate, the lower his risk of getting cancer.

In thirty-five of these studies the inverse associations were statistically significant. The evidence for benefit was strongest for cancers of the prostate, lung, and stomach. Data also suggested benefit for cancers of the pancreas, colon, rectum, esophagus, oral cavity, breast, and cervix. None of the studies showed adverse effects of high tomato intake.

Prostate cancer is the most common cancer and second leading cause of cancer mortality in men in the United States. Studies have suggested a potential benefit of tomato lycopene against the risk of prostate cancer, particularly in its more lethal forms. An 83 percent reduction of prostate cancer risk was observed in individuals with the highest plasma concentration of lycopene, compared to individuals with the lowest concentrations.[12]

I have been working very closely with a company named Wilson-Batiz to develop the most natural, pesticide-free tomatoes with very high concentrations of lycopene. These tomatoes are being sent to an FDA-approved lab in the United States to verify the high content of lycopene.

These tomatoes will be used as a part of the Oasis of Hope treatment program, but also they will soon be available in all major grocery stores. I applaud Wilson-Batiz for producing biologically functional foods without using chemicals and for introducing them to the general public.

Olive oil

Yet another functional food is olive oil, the principal source of fat in the Mediterranean diet. Think back to how many times olives and olive oil were mentioned in the Bible!

In more modern times, olive oil has been associated with health benefits that include the prevention of several varieties of cancers and the bolstering of the immune system. Olive oil contains several components that contribute to its overall therapeutic characteristics. And extra-virgin olive oil also contains a considerable amount of phenolic compounds, such as tyrosol and oleuropein, which exhibit antioxidant effects. Recent studies showed that phenolic compounds in olive oil help to suppress carcinogenesis.[13] It is so easy to incorporate things like olive oil into our diets. We all should do it!

Grapes

Grapes (another oft-mentioned biblical food) are known for their pharmacological properties. Grapes and wine contain high concentrations of a class of phytochemicals called polyphenols. Although their ability to protect from cancer has been well documented, the ways in which they do so, at the molecular level, are still unclear. However, it has been shown that grapes and grape extracts can be used as a chemopreventive agent against carcinogenesis, because:

- They inhibit oxidative stress and show a potent antiradical effect.

- They suppress cell proliferation and strongly inhibit tumor growth.

- They inhibit angiogenesis, and they strongly inhibit vascular endothelial growth factor, which inhibits the development of tumors and blood vessels.

- They tend to promote apoptosis (programmed cell death) in cancer cells.

Nuts

Almonds and other nuts confer health benefits despite their high fat content. The results from a recent study indicate that almond consumption may reduce colon cancer risk via at least one almond lipid-associated component.

Alfalfa

Alfalfa contains large amounts of chlorophyll, beta-carotene, and vitamin E. Alfalfa contains the nonprotein amino acid L-canavanine, which has antibacterial, antiviral, and antitumoral activities.

L-canavanine inhibited the in vitro growth of human pancreatic cancer and human melanoma. This nonprotein amino acid sensitized human colon and pancreatic cancer cells to Y-irradiation and enhanced the effect of 5-fluorouracil. It has also been shown that L-canavanine's antitumor mechanism of action is growth inhibition. Certain studies also indicate that L-canavanine, in combination with radiation, could have clinical potential in the treatment of cancer.

Juice

Freshly made vegetable juices offer excellent ways to receive nutrition. H. E. Kirschner, MD, explains why juices have such an impact on the restoration of the body:

> ...the power to break down the cellular structure of raw vegetables, and assimilate the precious elements they contain, even in the healthiest individual is only fractional—not more than 35 percent, and in the less healthy, down to 1 percent. In the form of juice, these same individuals assimilate up to 92 percent of these elements. It is a well-known fact that all foods must become liquid before they can be assimilated.[14]

It is also noteworthy that many people begin to have more digestive complaints as they age. This is due in part to a devitalized diet, but it is also because fewer enzymes are produced by the body. So, regardless of whether we partake of a relatively healthy diet or the standard American diet, we can have difficulty in digesting food as well as diminished nutrient assimilation.

When we juice, we bypass the digestive process. The fruit or vegetable has been broken down into a liquid form—the fiber has been removed—so nutrients are more easily absorbed and assimilated into the body, allowing it to utilize up to 92 percent of the available nutrients. It also is allowed to divert energy that would have been used for digestion into healing instead.

For those dealing with chronic conditions such as cancer, Hallelujah

Acres reports that consuming six to eight 8-ounce servings of freshly extracted vegetable juice daily is the quickest way to rebuild the body at the cellular level.

Omega-3 fatty acids

The omega-3 fatty acids are essential nutrients, and they are also fantastic disease fighters. Several thousand scientific publications testify to widespread agreement among medical professionals about the benefits of omega-3 fatty acids. For years, doctors have recognized the benefits of the Mediterranean diet, a diet rich in omega-3 fatty acids. Studies show that individuals who get a sufficient amount of these fatty acids in their diets experience a significantly lower risk of cancer mortality.

Some of the best sources of these acids are fish, plants, and oils. Fish are high in the omega-3 acids known as alpha-linolenic acid (ALA), eicosapentaenoic acid (EPA), and decosahexaenoic acid (DHA). Plants and oils contain the acid known as ALA. Plant sources relatively high in ALA content include nuts, seeds, and soybeans.

The content of ALA in soybean and canola oil is approximately 7.8 percent and 9.2 percent, respectively. Flaxseed oil is a particularly rich source of omega-3 fatty acids, mainly ALA, with an average content ranging from 57 percent to 69 percent, although it is not a commonly used food oil.

The following table illustrates the ALA content of a variety of sources.[15]

TERRESTRIAL PLANT SOURCES OF ALPHA-LINOLENIC ACID	
Source (100 g edible portion, raw)	**Alpha-linolenic acid (g) (ALA)**
Nuts and seeds	
• Almonds	0.4
• Flaxseed	22.8

TERRESTRIAL PLANT SOURCES OF ALPHA-LINOLENIC ACID	
Source (100 g edible portion, raw)	Alpha-linolenic acid (g) (ALA)
• Mixed nuts	0.2
• Peanuts	0.003
• Pecans	0.7
• Soybean kernels	1.5
• Walnuts, black	3.3
• Walnuts, English and Persian	6.8
Vegetables and legumes	
• Beans, navy and pinto, sprouted (cooked)	0.3
• Broccoli (raw)	0.1
• Cauliflower	0.1
• Lentils (dry)	0.2
• Lima beans (dry)	0.2
• Peas, garden (dry)	0.7
• Radish seeds, sprouted (raw)	3.2
• Soybeans, green (raw)	1.6
Vegetables and legumes	
• Soybeans (dry)	0.1
• Spinach (raw)	0.3
Grains	
• Barley, bran	0.3
• Corn, germ	0.3
• Oats, germ	1.4
• Rice, bran	0.2
• Wheat, bran	0.2
• Wheat, germ	0.7
Fruit	

TERRESTRIAL PLANT SOURCES OF ALPHA-LINOLENIC ACID	
Source **(100 g edible portion, raw)**	**Alpha-linolenic acid (g) (ALA)**
• Avocados (raw)	0.1
• Raspberries (raw)	0.1
• Strawberries (raw)	0.1

Chapter 10

TAKE ADVANTAGE OF NATURE'S PHARMACY

Cancer Beater #10

I AM A BIG FAN OF STORES LIKE WHOLE FOODS BECAUSE OF THEIR commitment to bringing pesticide-free fruits and vegetables to those who want them. I am also excited to see that the major grocery stores, and even large organizations like Costco, are featuring sections for produce that has been certified as having been grown organically.

In many of these places you can also find sections for vitamins, minerals, and herbal remedies. And in that area especially, you can find some very powerful anticancer agents. Scientists have identified specific healing substances in foods and have developed processes to extract these elements and concentrate them. But they are still food products. Let's talk about some of my favorite cancer-fighting products that come directly from nature.

Aged Garlic Extract

Several years ago I began using Kyolic Aged Garlic Extract as a natural antibiotic to treat ear infections. It worked wonders with my kids. Later on it earned a permanent spot in my medicine bag when I discovered its effectiveness as an antistress and antifatigue agent. When recent research demonstrated the role garlic plays in the health of the heart, a question occurred to me: could garlic offer similar benefits to cancer patients and people wishing to avoid it?

When I began to review the medical literature, I was thrilled to find that aged garlic extract constituents have been shown to be effective in inhibiting the growth and development of prostate cancer cells, melanoma cells, and neuroblastoma cells. In addition, these constituents slow the growth and development of carcinogen-induced tumors of the bladder, breast, colon, esophagus, stomach, and lung.

I was impressed with the extensive nature of these clinical studies. G. Li and collaborators found that two elements in aged garlic extract, called S-allyl cysteine (SAC) and S-allyl-mercaptocysteine, inhibit the growth and proliferation of breast cancer cells.[1] Better still, they also equip surrounding cells with tools they desperately need, like gluthathione-S-transferase and peroxidase. These are critical agents in cell detoxification and gene expression. In other words, they help cells get rid of the toxins that damage their ability to reproduce properly. Remember, when the gene expression process is compromised, the result is often a cancerous cell.

Much of garlic's activity derives from aliin and allicin or its immediate byproducts, such as S-allyl cysteine and S-allyl-mercaptocysteine found in aged garlic extracts. Garlic also contains selenium and tellurium.

Among aged garlic's other extract attributes are its anti-infection, antiaging, cardioprotective, and immune-enhancement properties. Additional research suggests that aged garlic extract might be useful for treating physiological aging and age-related memory disorders in humans.

I am not claiming that garlic can cure cancer, but I am saying that the constituents in aged garlic extract are important in combating carcinogens within the body. Clearly, garlic and aged garlic extract should be an integral part of your effort to equip your body to ward off disease. This is especially true considering the study conducted at Tufts University School of Medicine in Boston that concluded that aged garlic extract actually protects healthy cells against the oxidizing damage caused by chemotherapy.[2]

AHCC

Another way to bolster the immune system is through the use of active hexose correlated compound (AHCC), an extract obtained from several kinds of mushroom. Mushroom extracts are known to have immuno-modulating and antitumor effects. AHCC is very effective in strengthening and optimizing the capacity of the immune system.

The Oasis of Hope clinical research organization conducted a study comparing patients taking chemotherapy combined with AHCC and another group taking chemotherapy alone. One of the nasty side effects of chemotherapy is that it can severely depress the immune system. We found that AHCC truly protected the immune system from the depressing effects of chemotherapy.

AHCC can reduce the side effects of radiotherapy as well. AHCC also improves patients' quality of life by reducing nausea, increasing appetite, and decreasing anxiety. Furthermore, there are no side effects to taking AHCC as an immune-enhancing supplement.

Like melatonin, AHCC also stimulates the immune surveillance system. Cancer cells release several kinds of immune suppressive factors, which inhibit the body's ability to combat the disease. When the immune system is suppressed, something of a "chain reaction" occurs that results in the inhibition of the antitumor effects, which should come naturally to the body. The anticancer immune response fails when the production of killer cells fails. Thus, restoring the suppressed immune system is a very important part of cancer treatment, as is reversing any damage to it.

AHCC restores a depressed immune system and reverses damage by inhibiting the immune-suppressive factors produced by the cancer cells, increasing production of the cells that attack cancer, and stimulating the activity of the killer cells in particular. For this reason, AHCC is an important part of the well-rounded Oasis of Hope treatment program.

Coenzyme Q_{10}

Another powerful agent is CoQ_{10}, or coenzyme Q_{10}. This is a naturally occurring, fat-soluble substance that possesses vitamin-like properties. It is an essential component of the energy production process within our cells. However, while it is true that CoQ_{10} occurs naturally within the body, the levels decline as we age. If a person has high cholesterol, heart disease, or an addiction to cigarettes, these decreases can be significant. There is also clinical evidence linking cancer and immune system dysfunction to lowered levels of CoQ_{10}.

What does this substance do that is so important? It acts as an amazingly effective antioxidant by scavenging free radicals. This means that CoQ_{10} defends against the onset of cancer and destroys existing cancer. One study tracked patients with a variety of cancers. The study showed that 60 percent became cancer free during therapy with CoQ_{10}.[3]

Another report noted partial remission of breast cancer in over 10 percent of the "high-risk" patients studied. These patients were treated with CoQ_{10}. The same study also reported that the metastases of the cancer ceased during CoQ_{10} treatment. Both the regression of the primary tumor and the end of metastases in these cases are understood to be the result of the stimulating activity of coenzyme Q_{10} on the immune system.[4]

Doctors would be foolish not to equip their patients with this powerful, disease-fighting weapon.

Silymarin

Silymarin is a polyphenolic disease-fighting agent derived from milk thistle. Several studies have shown that silymarin is a very strong antioxidant, capable of scavenging both free radicals and reactive oxygen species, which results in a boost to cellular defense mechanisms.

For the last twenty years,[5] scientific researchers have also been studying the cancer chemopreventive and anticarcinogenic effects of silymarin.[6] These studies have shown that silymarin affords exceptional protection against cancers of the skin, prostate, breast, lung, colon, and bladder.

Silymarin can also significantly inhibit the growth of existing cancer as well. Recent studies have shown this inhibitory effect; researchers have concluded that silymarin can be an effective agent for both prevention and intervention. So how does it work?

One of the marks of cancer cells is the reckless abandon with which they reproduce. Silymarin inhibits this proliferation and alters the cell cycle progression in various types of cancer. When this happens, the cancer cells begin to suffer substantial apoptotic, or "programmed," death. The interruption to the cell cycle helps the body differentiate between healthy cells and cancer cells, thus enabling the body's immune system to target the cancer more effectively.

Let me confess that I am excited about the potential of silymarin because in the last couple of years, many clinical studies are concluding that silibinin, the main active agent in silymarin, is effective at combating colorectal cancer,[7] liver cancer,[8] prostate cancer,[9] bladder cancer,[10] and lung cancer.[11] Do you think all of my patients receive silymarin? You better believe they do!

Pancreatic Enzymes

There is a key difference between normal cells and tumor cells. Normal cells are programmed to grow rapidly in their juvenile state, but their programming changes as they mature, eventually dictating some function for the cells to serve within the body.

Tumor cells never mature. Their programming freezes in the juvenile state, and they continue to reproduce at an alarming rate, sending trophoblasts through the body's circulatory system in order to spread to other areas. So how do pancreatic enzymes address this problem?

Enzymes are essential biochemical units that play a necessary role in virtually all the functions of every organ system in the body. They are catalysts, substances that accelerate and precipitate the biochemical reactions that control the basic processes of life in each living organism. Each enzyme has a specific role in the body that no other enzyme can fill. To put it bluntly, life as we know it could not exist without enzymes.

Digestive enzymes are secreted along the gastrointestinal tract and break down foods, enabling the nutrients to be absorbed into the bloodstream for use in various bodily functions. Proteases (proteolytic enzymes), one of the three main categories of digestive enzymes, are found in the stomach juices, pancreatic juices, and intestinal juices. Proteolytic enzymes help to digest proteins.

Plant extracts with a high content of proteolytic enzymes have been used for years in traditional medicine. Besides proteolytic enzymes from plants, such as papain and bromelain obtained from papayas and pineapples respectively, "modern" enzyme therapy also includes proteolytic pancreatic enzymes, such as chymotrypsin, trypsin, pepsin, and pancreatin. Proteolytic enzymes are used primarily to aid the digestion and absorption of proteins contained in food. In addition to aiding digestion, proteolytic enzymes have analgesic, anti-inflammatory, antithrombotic, fibrinolytic, immune-modulating, and edema-reducing properties.

Results from recent research studies show that proteolytic enzymes can produce great benefits in cancer therapy by improving the patient's quality of life, reducing both the signs and symptoms of the disease and the adverse effects caused by radiotherapy and chemotherapy, and prolonging his or her survival time.[12]

Chapter 11

UNDERSTAND THE BRAIN-BODY CANCER CONNECTION

Cancer Beater #11

I T WAS CLOSE TO MIDNIGHT ON CHRISTMAS EVE, AND MY SISTERS, my brother, and I (Francisco Contreras), with our spouses by our sides, sat at the dinner table sharing with my parents the blessings that 1998 had brought us. The after-dinner testimonies, a tradition in the Contreras family, is my mother's highlight of every year. She is a very devout and committed Christian.

When my turn came to share, I looked into my mom's eyes and told her that I had decided to get closer to God. Her eyes got misty, a big smile came to her face, and "Amen!" was heard several times around the table. I think I also heard an "It's about time!" from one of my sisters.

The reason is that I am the black sheep of my family. All my brothers-in-law are ministers, only one of whom went to Bible college. The other three left professions in economics, administration, and oncology to serve the Lord, and now each one heads a large ministry in our home-town, Tijuana. My brother, also an oncologist, now dedicates most of his time to preaching the gospel in churches and on radio.

That Christmas Eve my mother, who dedicated me as a child to serve the Lord as a preacher, said with high expectations, "What are you planning to do?"

"I bought a Ducati 1098," I said.

"What is that?" she cried.

"A racing motorcycle," I said.

"How," she asked angrily, "will that get you closer to God?"

"Because, Mother, every time I drag my knee over the pavement while hugging a curve, my body, my soul, and my spirit shout in unison, 'Oh my God!'"

Aye, it was Francisco, the perennial jokester, who had to break the solemnity of the evening, giving all a chance to enjoy a good laugh. I have ridden motorcycles for many years, which includes amateur races and "track days." The rush I get from the combination of speed and fear makes my adrenals pump like crazy.

But I'm not entirely unique. There are lots of adrenaline junkies out there. Some get their "high" by doing dangerous stuff, but most get it by physically going "over the edge" through exercise, thus experiencing a natural high. It's natural, it's legal, and it's even godly.

God Designed Us to Experience Pleasure

Yes, even as He designed us to enjoy sex within marriage and thus to replenish the species, God also designed our bodies to derive pleasure from stressful situations, to develop endurance. It is important for us to understand this, especially given our goal of undermining cancer any way we can, so please bear with me in the next few pages. Some of this might seem like overly technical information, but I hope you find it as fascinating as I have.

Let's start by making it clear that adrenaline is not really the hormone responsible for the highs we commonly associate with it. Our brains release certain hormones known as *endorphins*, which cause euphoria with peak emotional and physical experiences. Thus, in reality we are *endorphin junkies*.

Endorphins belong to a class of biochemicals commonly referred to as *neurohormones*, which act by modifying the way in which nerve cells respond to transmitters.[1]

Endorphins and enkephalins are pain-blunting, pleasure-enhancing, opium- or morphine-like chemicals whose purpose, usually achieved in conjunction with adrenaline, is to make the body more effective, efficient, and ready for emergencies. They are intimately related to the "fight or flight" response described in the early twentieth century by Dr. Walter Cannon at Harvard Medical School.

This phenomenon may reveal itself at times via subtle, pleasurable, and physical manifestations, if you are able to recognize what you're looking at, as I do when I race motorcycles. The same phenomenon can be equally terrifying when the threat cannot be completely recognized or is too great to handle, such as an attack from a wild animal. Either way, stress thus becomes part of how we experience the world about us.

Dr. William Glasser calls this "the quality world,"[2] meaning that it's the core of our lives. We continually modify it so that it reflects what we want now. We build it, starting shortly after birth, from all we have perceived that feels very good. What feels very good is anything we do that satisfies us. Or, in the case of addictions, anything that *seems* to satisfy one or more of five basic needs built into our genetic structure: the need for survival, love and belonging, power, freedom, and fun.[3]

Mechanics of "Fight or Flight"

When confronted with a life-threatening event, we go into a high level of "body alarm reaction," and the hypothalamus in the base of our brains starts a cascade of biochemical responses that activate the *limbic* and *immune* systems within nanoseconds. The body will be instructed to hit, duck, run, or fake death to avoid being a target.

The neurochemical portion of this cascade begins in the hypothalamus and the pituitary gland, targeting the adrenal cortex and producing hyper brainwave activity, which causes increased vigilance, concentration, and alertness. Our pupils dilate so we can see as much as possible of our surroundings, and both our facial expressions and body stances instantly change.

At the same time, the palms of our hands get sticky so we can hold on if we have a weapon. Our skin chills, our hair stands, and extra blood floods into our muscles to prepare us for a burst of action. Our breathing speeds up even as our airways dilate, which allows the air to move in and out of the lungs more quickly. Our hearts race and our blood pressure skyrockets, infusing our bodies with oxygen.

Blood vessels of the organs most directly involved in either exercise or fighting off danger—including skeletal muscles, cardiac muscles, the liver, and adipose tissue—dilate to allow faster flow of blood. Our blood glucose level rises, and our livers get busy metabolizing glycogen to glucose, while adipose tissue splits triglycerides to fatty acids, both of which are used by muscle fiber to generate energy for quick fuel. In addition, cholesterol levels go up because cholesterol is a precursor to hormone production, and it also thickens blood so that, in case of injury, clotting will be faster and more efficient.

The immune system is called instantly to full alert. Nonessential physiological processes switch off. The blood vessels of nonessential organs, such as the reproductive system, the kidneys, and the gastrointestinal tract, constrict and often even void their contents.

Later, after the hazardous situation passes, the parasympathetic nervous system halts all secretions and turns off all hormone-inducing glands. At that point the goal is to achieve homeostasis and bring all the body's organs and functions back to normal as quickly as possible.[4]

Therefore, if we successfully fight, flee, or play dead, what follows is a "cool down" period that could involve shaking, gasps or sighs, shuddering, or other forms of release that can often lead to exhaustion before the body regains its balance and achieves equilibrium. Thus the physical arousal associated with fight or flight cannot be sustained indefinitely.

The beauty of this mechanism is unquestionable, but our modern lifestyle repeatedly presents it with tremendous challenges for which it really was not designed. Here are the two most common causes.

- First, a life-threatening situation is not necessary to unleash the neurochemical cascade. *The perception of danger alone is sufficient*, and we've been conditioned to perceive imaginary threats on many fronts. For example, all physicians know that the mere sight of their white coats will cause an immediate rise in blood pressure and cholesterol levels in perfectly healthy patients, because so many patients expect their doctors to tell them things they do not wish to hear.

- Second, when the threat lasts longer than the few minutes that this response was designed for (such as a diagnosis of cancer that requires the patient to confront the threat of death, real or perceived, not in the next few minutes, but in weeks, months, and even years), the fight or flight system gets no chance to turn off and rest, provoking a completely new set of biochemical reactions.

At the International Society for Neuro-immunomodulation Conference in November 1996, Dr. Philip Gold of the National Institute of Mental Health said:

> In many people their hormones, such as cortisol, turn on and stay on for a long time. If you are in danger, cortisol is good for you. But if it becomes unregulated, it can produce disease. In extreme cases, this hormonal state destroys appetite, cripples the immune system, shuts down processes that repair tissue, blocks sleep, and even breaks down bone.[5]

How Does "Fight or Flight" Affect Cancer Patients?

Cancer patients who once tended to view life as a series of possibilities—a spectrum of colors—may begin to experience their world in blacks and whites, as either/or, us/them, or right/wrong with no gradations or in-betweens. Time becomes an enemy because quick decisions need to be made, one after the other.

The patient's sense of listening will also be skewed. The ability to prioritize goes out the window when overwhelming stress gives everything number one status. This results in immobility, confusion, and the inability to make even the smallest decisions. It also leads to seemingly random outbursts of emotion, depression, and even the kind of anger that looks for someone or something to blame.

If the fight or flight response system is not told to stand down and revert to a noncrisis situation, it will continue to maintain a high alert status in the body. Stress maintains that alert status. Prolonged stress of any kind will eventually deplete the adrenal glands and cause depression of the immune system and possible tumor growth.[6]

Beyond all the above, the supposed "objectivity" so prized in our modern culture (even though it is sometimes no more than a legalistic response to unspecified threats of lawsuits) has created a culture of terror for cancer patients. Doctors are expected, on both ethical and legal grounds, to disclose the complete diagnosis and prognosis to their patients, based on known statistics.[7]

However, even though feel-good approaches and patient cheering usually are discouraged and qualified as unscientific, new and not-so-new data continue to challenge this position.[8]

So What Can You Do?

In 1999, scientists at the University of Alabama in Huntsville reported to the national meeting of the American Chemical Society, the world's largest scientific society, that large doses of vitamin C can prevent illness by alleviating the body's normal response to stress.

The study showed that vitamin C reduced the levels of stress hormones in the blood and also reduced other typical indicators of physical and emotional stress, such as loss in body weight, enlargement of the adrenal glands, and reduction in the size of the thymus gland and the spleen. In addition, vitamin C treatment elevated the levels of circulating IgG antibody, the body's principal defense against systemic infection.

In the control group—that is, rats that were not subjected to stress—vitamin C increased the production of IgG antibody to a somewhat higher level than it did in the stressed rats. Consequently, animals—and perhaps people—who are under emotional stress might require higher doses of vitamin C to protect immune function.

Many reports in the medical literature have demonstrated vitamin C's immune system-boosting capacity. For example, it boosted immune function in a test group of elderly women. It also reduced the incidence of stress-related upper-respiratory infections in marathon runners.

Our prehistoric ancestors probably consumed large amounts of vitamin C in a tropical diet rich in fruits. Why should we not do the same? The researchers conclude:

> ...the physiological constitution we have inherited may require doses far larger than the present RDA to keep us healthy under varying environmental conditions, including stress.[9]

Have a Chocolate Pepper!

Endorphin secretion may also be triggered by the consumption of certain foods, such as chocolate and chili peppers.

Indeed, the characteristic increase in bodily endorphin levels caused by chocolate could explain why we often turn to it as a comfort food in times of stress. Chocolate is by far the most popular endorphin-producing food on the earth.

Known by the Aztecs as the food of the gods, chocolate is derived from cacao beans that were revered by the Aztecs, who believed that eating chocolate would confer wisdom and vitality. Chocolate contains more than three hundred different compounds, including anandamide, a chemical that mimics marijuana's soothing effects on the brain. It also contains chemical compounds such as flavonoids (which are also found in wine) that have antioxidant properties and reduce serum cholesterol.

Although the combined psychochemical effects of these compounds on the central nervous system are poorly understood, the production of endorphins is believed to contribute to the renowned "inner glow" experienced by dedicated chocolate lovers. But as with red wine, moderation is the key. Consuming more than 50 grams a day is not recommended.

Many popular ethnic foods, including Tex-Mex, Mexican, Cajun, Indian, Chinese (especially Szechuan), and Thai, are renowned for their spiciness. The resulting endorphin rush keeps diners coming back for more. Chili peppers provide a stimulating heat and "bite" that increases the body's production of endorphins.

Chili peppers are not all created equal: red peppers are generally more pungent than green ones, and hotter chilies grow at higher altitudes and warmer temperatures. Chilies also release their heat differently. Some are experienced as "hot" immediately, or their pungency is released over time; some chilies cause a burning sensation in the back of the throat, while others affect the tongue or the lips.

And while chili peppers vary as to flavor, texture, and color, they all provide important vitamins and minerals, including vitamin A, calcium, and vitamin C. Moreover, due to the endorphin release associated with chili peppers, they have been utilized in various kinds of medical treatments, especially as part of therapy for chronic pain, and are sometimes considered an aphrodisiac.

I'm sure this is one of the reasons why Mexicans have such a low incidence of cancer and are so warm and happy.

Chapter 12

COPE WITH STRESS

Cancer Beater #12

I (DANIEL KENNEDY) GREW UP IN THE 1970s, WHEN CORNY VARIETY shows were the "in" thing. I watched more *Lawrence Welk*, *Donny & Marie*, and *Hee Haw* than anyone should ever have to endure. Nonetheless, one of my favorite bits from *Hee Haw* came with Buck Owens and Roy Clark singing about their deep despair, gloom, and agony. They said that their only luck was bad luck. I love that. And in the 1980s, The Police sang about all the awful things that happened to the singer: bit by his own dog, a son that "turned out gay," and a runaway teenage daughter. Wow.

In more recent times the catch phrase taken to new highs (or lows!) by Donald Trump, "You're fired," connects with human fears and stressors once again.

We humans are a brooding, depressed, anxious, fearful, hope-deficient race. I am generalizing, true, but try to tell me that you've never had a stress headache or felt your heart race because of a deadline. Tell me you've never felt overwhelmed, wanting only to escape whatever pressures you were feeling at the moment.

Heavy negative emotions are part of life. We have been designed to experience them for a specific reason. They are reactions to threatening circumstances, and their purpose is to help us cope and survive. They are red flags that signal our body to react.

However, in addition to the physical aspects outlined by Dr. Contreras, your ability to manage negative emotions and promote positive emotions has a powerful influence on whether you develop cancer and on your success in reversing it.

So how are you doing in terms of stress management? Clearly, life is more stressful today than it was fifty years ago. In addition to cell phones, fax machines, and pagers, we now have text messaging and e-mail to contend with every day. All these things facilitate instant communication, but we never have a moment to ourselves. Have you seen the magazine ads that show laptop owners using their computers at the beach? Who wants to go to Hawaii just to continue working?

Aside from the high-paced life, much of the world has been affected by the events of 9/11. Every day, it seems, we read reports about threats of more attacks in other cities, using biological weapons, poisons, and even nuclear "dirty" bombs.

One obvious result of all this is that depression, once thought to be experienced only by those at midlife or older, is now plaguing our youth. A number of researchers explain that adolescents suffer from existential dread. In an article from February 2004 about a young man who committed suicide in Tampa, Florida, the reporter interviewed teens who seemed to understand why the youth had taken his life because they had experienced the same kind of unhappiness. According to the article, "Each [teen] expressed feelings of hopelessness about the future."[1]

To add to all these stresses, today's young people look around and note that the adults are all stressed out too and not very happy with what they've achieved. *Maybe this helps explain why the mean age for a diagnosis of cancer has decreased dramatically over the last twenty years.* When my grandfather started treating cancer patients in the 1960s, most of his patients were older than sixty years of age. It was rare for him to have a patient younger than fifty.

Today, more than half of our patients are younger than forty-five.

Why? One major reason is that our bodies pay the price of unmanaged physical and emotional stress. *Stress is one of cancer's major strong-holds.* Manage that, and you undermine cancer.

Dr. Contreras has already discussed several things you can do of a physical nature. In the next few chapters, we will provide easy and effective ways to get your *psychological and emotional* stress under control as well.

Your Mind—a Powerful Healing Agent

The four-minute mile had been the impossible dream of every world-class runner for many years, until everything changed on May 6, 1954, at a track meet in the United Kingdom. As a young man from the United States completed the first lap, his heart leapt with excitement as he heard the time: 57.5 seconds. He wasn't in first place, but he was pushing the leader. His time at the second lap was 1 minute, 58 seconds. But at the third lap, his time was 3 minutes, 0.07 seconds, and he was still in second place. How could he possibly run the final lap in less than 59 seconds?

Roger Bannister told what happened when he realized how close he was, and yet how far away:

> I had a moment of mixed joy and anguish, when my mind took over. It raced well ahead of my body and drew my body compel-lingly forward. I felt that the moment of a lifetime had come. There was no pain, only a great unity of movement and aim. The only reality was the next two hundred yards of track under my feet.[2]

Bannister defied many years of "running wisdom" that day, breaking through the tape at 3 minutes, 59.4 seconds. Amazingly, his tremendous belief not only helped him accomplish the impossible himself, but it also pulled two other runners through in less than four minutes as well! It took these three men to show others that it was possible. People all over the world now run the mile in less than four minutes.

Take Another Look

Let's look again at the beginning of the Bannister quote: "I had a moment of mixed joy and anguish, when my mind took over." One of your most important assets in the fight against cancer is your mind. It is absolutely critical for you to consider how you think about cancer, especially about having it yourself.

Having worked with thousands of cancer patients, I can attest that patients who state that they are going to die of cancer almost always do. Patients who say that they are going to beat cancer markedly improve their chances of survival. Indeed, even the pessimists who beat the odds have usually had positive people around them—wives or husbands, mothers, or friends who remained optimistic and encouraging no matter what.

Many things are beyond your control, but only you can decide what your attitude will be.

If you have cancer, I encourage you to tackle the problem head-on and decide that, no matter what happens, cancer won't triumph over you emotionally. If we just give up, cancer wins the ultimate battle, the one fought over the human spirit, not the body. If we fight with a passion that will not give up against any odds, we can turn the tables.

Max Factor's son was a patient of Oasis of Hope before I started working here. Donald Factor was one of those people with a winning attitude. Though his lab results indicated that he most certainly would die, he never accepted that possibility. He would not accept defeat. Twenty-six years later he still lives cancer free. He visits each year, and he has taught everyone at the hospital a lot about the power of the human spirit.

I am not telling you to live in denial. In fact, studies indicate that denial is counterproductive. Cancer is a serious illness that has to be acknowledged. But I am saying that you should not declare that you are dying of cancer, because your body will believe you and obey. Death does not need any help from you. It will come soon enough all by itself. You do not need to usher it in. Instead, focus all your energies and attention on living.

I like what Patch Adams shared in the foreword he wrote to *The Hope of Living Cancer Free*:

I know we have a world panic about cancer. But the worst cancer is being alive and not enjoying it, not feeling gratitude, not loving, not living. It is not the dying that is really a big deal; it is the dying in life that is bad. To go around thinking, "Life is a struggle, life is terrible and then you die," that's the worst cancer.[3]

That is why a lot of people who get a cancer diagnosis end up being thankful, because it wakes them up to life. This happens all the time. Cancer is so surreal it becomes a blessing. People begin to appreciate the simple things, like flowers and a glass of lemonade.

The question about cancer should not be if we can get rid of it. Eventually this fabulous machine of a body will break down, and each of us will die of something. We will never overcome death on this side of eternity. The real question is whether or not we can recognize where we really are when cancer hits and move beyond all that to experience life as fully as possible in the time we have left.

We all know people whose cancer is never more than a nuisance. Even if it eventually kills them, they enjoy life while they are alive. If you love your life and live it in absolute fullness, then *whenever and however you die*, you will have lived while you were alive.

That makes it all worthwhile, whether a cure comes or not.

That's also why, in addition to addressing the physical causes of cancer, we need to address the emotional factors as well. I don't think we fully understand how much of a role negative emotions can play in incubating cancer. Hostility, depression, anxiety, loneliness, unforgiveness, lack of love—all these have negative power.

Death is the final chapter. It should not be feared, but eventually it should be embraced. Meanwhile, no one wants to die before his or her time. So don't! Take Patch's advice and start living. Do not take a cancer diagnosis as a death sentence. Take back your life and make every day count.

Let's talk about specific ways to do that.

Identity Crisis

It distresses me to see so many who are diagnosed with cancer go through an identity crisis. Maybe the person was a schoolteacher, wife, mother, choir member, or avid snow skier. The moment she was diagnosed, in her mind, she became a cancer patient above all else.

No one should ever be reduced to that level. You are still everything you have ever been; the only "new" thing is that you are now dealing with a health challenge called cancer. Get on with all your important things, and make lots of plans for your future. Get to your doctor appointments and take your medications, but make that a part of your day and not your whole life.

I have met many patients who have made surviving cancer their mission in life. I believe that overcoming cancer is a fine goal, but it should be a means to a greater end.

When I am counseling patients, I always ask them, "If you were to make a deal with God and He cured you of cancer, what would you do in return?" Many people will say, "I would start raising funds to help others." Or, "I will start spending quality time with my child." Then I suggest, "Why not start your new mission now?" You don't have to wait until you are cancer free to live a meaningful life.

The main concept here is that if you think of yourself as a cancer patient who is dying, guess what? That's what you will be. If you think of yourself as a valuable person living a meaningful life who also just happens to be dealing with cancer, that is what you will be.

It is also extremely important for you to "release" cancer in emotional and spiritual terms. *Do not accept ownership of the disease.* If you catch yourself saying, "My cancer is such-and-such," stop and rephrase. Call it *the* cancer, never *yours*.

This might seem like a strange example, but think of your own children. When the kids get to be twenty-one or so, it's time to let them move out on their own. Sometimes it takes a lot of letting go, but you have to do it for your own good. And for theirs as well, of course, but that's not my point.

Let cancer go! Don't hold on to it and be its doting parent. Don't scold it, don't dress it, and don't take it to soccer practice. In emotional terms, *kick it out of the house!*

Most people develop entirely new relationships with their kids after they leave home. That's their reward for doing the right thing. Do the same with cancer, except that you don't have to be its friend! Even as it stays inside your body, *let it live on the other side of town.*

Find a Miracle

Here's another important concept. *Find a miracle, or something meaningful, that happens around you even as you deal with cancer.* Being cured of cancer is not the only good thing you can identify with and experience. Many great things happen to people *after* they are diagnosed.

Chapter 13

THINK POSITIVE THOUGHTS

Cancer Beater #13

As a young teenager I (Daniel Kennedy) once went roller-skating with a church youth group, which included a girl I was eager to impress. Naturally I was convinced that something disastrous would therefore happen, only partly because I'd never gone roller-skating before!

We arrived at the rink, and I immediately broke into a sweat. I wanted this girl to think I was cool, not to see me using my head as a battering ram. My "friends"—and I use that term loosely—assured me that everything would be fine, that I would catch on to this new thing in no time at all.

I rented a pair of skates the color of baby puke and strapped them to my feet. I moved toward the opening to the rink, where scores of young boys and girls now swirled gracefully in a perpetual left-hand turn. I took a few tentative steps and I was off! I was not the picture of perfection, but for a few seconds I actually managed to look coordinated. Then I saw her.

She was at the wall about twenty yards up, looking my direction. I thought, "Don't fall, don't fall, don't fall." So, of course, I fell. I'm not even sure what happened, but there is probably a very humorous "flap-flap" dance named after me somewhere.

Self-Fulfilling Prophecy

I mention all this to illustrate the concept of the self-fulfilling prophecy. What we worry about often *does* happen because our anxiety brings it about. But while a self-fulfilling prophecy can help cause disaster, as it did for me that day, it can also bring about a blessing.

What a person hopes will happen actually *can* happen; our expectations can make it so.

Many people think of the body as the primary battleground for cancer, but I believe the real war is fought in the heart and mind of the patient. Fear of cancer makes a person believe he will die, and if he is fully convinced, his likelihood of survival shrinks. Negative emotions actually have a devastating physiological impact.

Yet if a patient is freed of fear, healing becomes much more likely. That freedom also opens the door to other meaningful experiences not affected by advance or remission of the cancer. The person who experiences such freedom is victorious no matter what the lab results say.

Here are stories about three cancer victors. Two are still living while one has passed away, but all three defeated cancer. The words in quotations were spoken or written by the patients themselves.

Dee

"Twelve years ago I was diagnosed with breast cancer. I was devastated and shocked. First of all, I couldn't believe this could happen to me. I had never been sick, not even with a cold, and I had always considered myself to be a very healthy person. Immediately, I had a decision to make—did I want to live, or did I want to die? My choice was obvious.

"Fortunately, the first part of my journey took me to Oasis of Hope Hospital, where I met and became a patient of Dr. Francisco Contreras. Immediately my life was touched by a staff and an environment that reassured and comforted me. They offered me peace and healing. I was treated in not only a professional way but also as a personal family member.

"Oasis's focus was on the whole patient, not just the disease. With the assistance of Dr. Contreras and the hospital staff, I learned how to take charge of my life. This was the real journey, the journey to healing. I soon became an avid student of nutrition and quickly learned how to apply the best of science and the best of nature to my personal life. I also learned that health is the most valuable possession in life.

"Cancer is the ultimate battle. It forces you to fight for your life. Cancer does not discriminate. Only a few years ago, cancer was referred to as a condition too awful to discuss. However, knowledge is a powerful weapon. Survivors know cancer can be conquered, and they learn to speak the language of warfare. They truly have fought an enemy within—not simply the intruding cells but denial, anger, and despair as well.

"Many cancer survivors consider the disease to have been a gift in a horrible package, a message too dire to ignore: life, which is indeed fleeting and precious, is a miracle and a gift from God. I know hope is the most powerful medicine of all. Illness is an opportunity for growth, and the healing part comes from the ability to deal with whatever illness is troubling you. It's all about finding peace of mind.

"How did an experience so tragic bring good into my life? It was a lesson to teach me where to turn in a crisis. It pulled me into a dark valley, dropping me along the way—forcing me to rest and learn to trust. Psalm 46:10 says, 'Be still and know that I am God.'

"He was in control. I emerged on the mountaintop, in the same world but with a different appreciation of life and a closer relationship with my Savior. Yes, I touched the rose and felt the thorn. I've seen my life go from 'vision to victory.'

"We cannot tell what may happen to us in the strange medley of life, but we can decide what happens within us how we take it and what we do with it. That's what really counts in the end—how to take the raw stuff of life and make it a thing of worth and beauty. That is the test of living. The magic of life can never end, for it's filled with all of life's greatest gifts—our family and friends.

"If you are struggling with illness, remember the importance of a positive mental attitude, and do not give up hope. Arm yourself with knowledge about your illness, and become an active participant in your treatment plans."

Jack

Jack Riley was a senior triathlete. He entered races that involved swimming, biking, and running. A triathlon is a grueling sport even for the young, but Jack had begun in midlife. A former drinker, smoker, and junk-food advocate, Jack traded his bourbon glass for running shoes. Yet, despite his late start, Jack competed in 644 marathons and triathlons.

After being diagnosed and treated for prostate cancer, Jack became a hero in Alamo, California, when he was tapped to carry the Olympic torch in San Francisco during the torch relay. But he didn't stop there—he passed the official flame on to the next runner, dipped his foot in the Pacific, and then ran, biked, and swam 3,300 miles to the Olympic stadium in Atlanta, his *personal* Olympic torch in hand. He then continued on to the Atlantic Ocean.

In 1997 he ran, biked, and swam 1,700 miles from Vancouver, Canada, to Tijuana, Mexico. Jack's runs took him through 300 towns. Through the media, more than 15 million people were made aware of his quest.

But for Jack, none of the publicity really mattered. Everywhere he went he visited children's cancer centers, helping to cheer the children he found there, giving them courage to fight their own battles against cancer. These were the true highlights of Jack's trips.

In the last phase of his life, Jack still concentrated on living. When I asked Jack what the motivation for his transnational triathlons had been, he replied, "I am a competitor. I guess it is in my blood. If I can do this for a good cause, well, that's what life is all about. I will do this as long as I can, as long as God gives me the physical, mental, and emotional ability. I see cancer as a competitor too, but I don't dwell on it. I dwell on my own performance, which is in the hands of God."

On Jack's third and final triathlon of hope, he made it from the Pacific

Ocean through thirteen cities in California and Arizona. At the New Mexico border his body gave out, though his spirit never did. Jack Riley passed away on July 1, 1998. His wife told me that he died the way he wanted to, serving others and fighting for a cure.

Jack Riley is still a role model for those with a cancer challenge, because he kept a positive attitude. In a day when it's difficult to find a hero, Jack showed courage, commitment, love, integrity, and focus. The memory of Jack motivates me to do something meaningful with my own life. When I feel challenged and overwhelmed, I think of Jack. He had cancer, and yet he still accomplished so much.

William

One day we were having a prayer service at the hospital. One of our pastors approached a patient named William, who was there on a follow-up visit. When William was asked if he wanted prayer for healing, he responded, "I don't need to be healed of cancer. I have already been blessed more than I deserve. I have been married to my lovely wife for fifty years. Plus, some wonderful things have come about since I was diagnosed. A number of my friends who didn't know Christ now do because they started to spend more time with me, and we would pray together.

"Also, I have three children, all of whom had broken marriages. The kids started to get together to pray, and now two of those marriages have been restored, and I am waiting for the third one to get back together with his wife."

Many people feel that anything less than a cure is a failure. They seem to feel that cancer looks like a winner anytime a person dies of it. But my patients have demonstrated to me just how incorrect that point of view is. I encourage them to search for meaning through the experience and look for the hidden miracles in the process. That is what William did.

I also ask people to expand their definition of what a valid outcome would look like. For many patients, that valid outcome becomes the enjoyment of many years of quality living even though the cancer persists.

"The Patient Died, but the Treatment Worked"

As I shared in the introduction, I (Francisco Contreras) will never forget the time I accompanied my father to the famed Memorial Sloan-Kettering Cancer Center in New York to share successful case studies with leading oncologists from around the world. My father put up a patient's diagnostic chest X-ray alongside a post-treatment X-ray. The tumor was still there. One of the oncologists stood up and said, "That's not a successful case."

He left the room and returned with comparative X-rays of one of his patients. The diagnostic X-ray showed a tumor, and the post treatment X-ray did not. My father congratulated the doctor and asked how the patient was doing. The oncologist stated with no remorse, "The patient died, but the treatment was successful."

My father humbly pointed out that even though cancer was still present in his patient, the X-rays had been taken ten years apart, and the patient continued to live and work with the cancer completely under control. I was dumbfounded when the oncologist told my father that it was a nice story but that only objective results, such as measurable tumor reduction, constituted a valid outcome.

Patients who have found ways to peacefully coexist with cancer would disagree. Controlling cancer is also a valid outcome. For many such patients, success can be defined as outliving their prognoses by months and sometimes even years. This outcome becomes even more mean-ingful, and thus more valuable, when patients truly begin to live and to amass meaningful moments.

I never imagined that two decades later an oncologist who was trained at Memorial Sloan-Kettering would partner with us as we opened up Oasis of Hope in Southern California. He is forward thinking and under-stands how wrapping care around a patient is what a patient needs.

It is always wonderful to see people come to terms with life and the people around them. My father received a letter from a woman telling him that her husband had passed away, but she had much to be grateful for. While he was being treated, he found peace and love, and he was able to forgive his father for childhood abuse.

After that he lived six more months, during which his wife said he was a new man. He had never been affectionate with his children, but in those six months his girls learned what it was to have a loving father. The man was not cured, and he did not coexist for long with the cancer, but he experienced life in a new way and gave his family many wonderful gifts.

Quality of life is much more important than quantity. You can kick the feet out from under cancer if you can adapt your "great expectations." If a cure is the only acceptable resolution for you, you just might miss out on some incredible blessings.

Step 1: Reframing Negative Thoughts

Do you remember the story about the optimist and the pessimist who were also identical twins? They were genetic equals but psychological opposites. A psychologist wanted to find out why, so he put the pessimist in a room full of toys and the optimist in a room full of manure.

Five minutes later, when the counselor opened the first door, he found the pessimist huddled in a corner, weeping bitterly. "I know these toys are not mine, and I can't take them with me," the child cried.

The psychologist then looked in on the optimist, who was digging frantically through the manure with a huge smile on his face. "There must be a pony in there somewhere!" he said.

How we process our "world" determines who we are and how we experience life. The Book of Proverbs says that we are how we think. This is a profound concept, suggesting that our worldview, our orientation, our perceptions, and our coping strategies are all exceedingly important.

When I (Daniel Kennedy) was a teenager, I was always depressed. Why? Because I believed that whenever things seemed to be going well, disaster was just around the corner. I didn't want to express happiness or get too excited, because I truly believed that it would increase the likelihood that something bad would happen.

Why? Well, I had a very happy childhood until my mother died in a plane crash when I was eleven. My devastation convinced me that it would be *too risky* ever to feel happy again.

But even for a person like me, who once had such an extremely negative emotional paradigm, there is hope. Through counseling and a personal relationship with God, I saw my personal paradigm shift a full 180 degrees. Now, I believe that *good* things are going to happen! And when tough times come, I know they will last only a while. I agree with the psalmist who wrote that troubles may last for the night, but joy comes in the morning.

Our Automatic Thoughts Really Matter

In like manner, many different factors can influence how a person views cancer. It might be difficult for someone to believe they can overcome cancer if they saw it kill both their grandfather and their mother. Conversely, it's often easier for someone whose brother survived cancer to believe he or she can survive as well.

If a person is able to generate healthy, positive thoughts *automatically*, he or she is emotionally structured for success. Their probability of survival automatically increases, and a meaningful life, no matter how long it lasts, becomes much more likely.

What do I mean by automatic thoughts? These are the cognitive responses that come as automatic responses to given stimuli, not as products of contemplation. All patients have quite a few automatic thoughts about the various aspects of cancer and treatment, and most of these are negative thoughts for most people.

For example, when a person has a malignancy, any little pain or discomfort will automatically be associated with the illness. A patient may feel a pain in his or her back and think, "Oh, no, maybe I have a tumor in my spine." Needless to say, millions of healthy people have back pain every day, but they don't automatically assume that they have tumors.

Negative Thoughts Have Physical Consequences!

Negative thoughts produce negative emotions, which in turn depress the immune system. Many clinical studies demonstrate the direct cause/effect correlation, but one such study put it in perhaps the simplest terms of all: "If you're sad or blue, you're more likely to get sick."[1]

Through interviewing hundreds of cancer patients, I have found that most go through six separate emotional stages before they reach number seven, which represents the goal.

In a moment I want to talk about a very effective cognitive restructuring technique you can use to avoid the above pitfalls. But first, let's take a look at the negative emotions commonly experienced by people who have cancer.

1. The first stage is *shock*. Most people have no idea what it is like to sit in a doctor's office and have him look them in the eye and say, "I am very sorry to tell you this, but you have cancer." Breaking that news is never a pleasant experience. It is like chaining a five-hundred-pound weight onto a person's leg and pushing them to the edge of a pier. The news generates shock because it is usually unexpected. Surprisingly, few people share the news with loved ones until the shock wears off, yet solid support structure of family and friends to rally around them is vital.

2. The second stage, *denial*, can often accompany the first. Facing one's own mortality can be so difficult that many people, at first, are unable to acknowledge this new reality. Some will even accuse their physician of incompetence, openly or secretly. They may adopt a cavalier attitude and think, "This isn't that big of a deal!" or, "I can beat this thing easy!" But it is incredibly dangerous to underestimate the seriousness of the threat cancer poses. The first step in getting a patient into a comprehensive treatment

program is helping him acknowledge what he is up against.

3. The third stage, *fear*, can also accompany the first. Seconds after hearing the cancer diagnosis, some people are overwhelmed with fear, which is often twofold. The patient experiences fear of death and also fear of the suffering associated with both cancer itself and conventional treatments. I have seen strong evidence that fear is one of cancer's most powerful strongholds—it can literally fuel the progression of the tumor. Helping a patient fully embrace the hope of healing is a critical step in establishing positive emotional health.

4. The fourth stage, *grief*, comes when the reality of the situation has had time to settle. Sometimes in the middle of a very successful treatment program the patient is suddenly overwhelmed with sadness. The possibility of missing out on certain things, especially the lives of loved ones, can be a crushing reality. While this emotion is completely normal, it becomes counterproductive if it goes unaddressed. Grief can become so intense it can cause people to isolate themselves from the very support structure they so desperately need. Often, patients will close themselves off to others in an effort to spare the people they love pain and suffering. However, the emotional burden of a fight with cancer must be shared, because it is too intense for anyone to bear alone.

5. The fifth stage, *anger*, often comes after the patient is fully engaged in the battle. Patients find themselves asking, "Why me, God?" Many are tempted to suppress these questions as inappropriate, but I couldn't disagree more. In fact, I firmly believe that obtaining the answer to that question is extremely important. On the other hand, swal-

lowing the question will only breed resentment and will cripple a patient's faith.

6. The sixth stage is connected to the fifth. If people attempt to work through the "why me" question without support, they may experience feelings of *guilt* or inadequacy. They may think, "I deserve this. This is my fault." Or, "I'm not getting better because I lack faith." Again, these feelings are normal and understandable, but dangerous if not worked through fully. Patients need help in coming to terms with the fragile nature of life and the fine line between health and illness.

7. The seventh stage, *acceptance* and resolve, is the goal. When patients reach this stage, they have reached a positive emotional state that does not compromise their chances for healing. They have accepted their situation and have decided to be proactive in seeking a solution.

The beginning of restructuring the way you think about cancer and related subjects requires you to identify your negative automatic thoughts. It is also important to know what types of issues can provoke negative emotions.

Reframing Negatives

The best cognitive restructuring technique I know of is called reframing. When you catch yourself thinking or stating something negative, write it down. Then think about it and come up with a way to "reframe" or reinterpret what you thought was bad as something positive. Then write your new positive thought next to the negative thought and start working to replace the negative with the positive.

After that, each time you catch yourself starting to have the negative thought, say, "Stop." Then, in an audible voice, repeat the positive thought. After a while you will begin to internalize the change, and the positive thought will become automatic.

Here are examples of negative automatic thoughts. Try to think up some positive thoughts and write them in on the right side—for example, just to get started you might consider writing, "I am living with cancer," after the first entry.

Negative Automatic Thoughts	Positive Automatic Thoughts
I am dying of cancer.	
I will not respond to treatment.	
I am a burden to others.	
I am of no use to anyone now.	
God is punishing me.	
I must have done something to deserve this.	
Others can recover, but I probably won't.	

How did you do? Once you get the hang of it, you can rid yourself of any thought not likely to help you overcome cancer.

In group sessions at Oasis of Hope and at conferences, I like to do this reframing exercise via audience participation. At one such workshop for a women's group in London, I started to present negative thoughts and asked people to come up with positive replacements. Some great statements came from the crowd, but one stopped me right in my tracks.

My negative statement was, "I only have a 5 percent probability of survival." A woman in the audience immediately responded, "I am not a statistic."

Absolutely! Great! Who wants to be a statistic? Who wants to own a disease? Who wants to be a victim? That one said it all!

Have you ever discovered that being a pessimist brings about good outcomes? Has worrying brought good things to you? Automatic negative thoughts do not help either. Reframing negative thoughts into positive thoughts and replacing the bad with the good will eventually restructure your thought processes so that you can actually think in a healthy manner. Keep practicing this technique; it will help.

Chapter 14

SURROUND YOURSELF WITH POSITIVE FRIENDS

Cancer Beater #14

OVER THE YEARS I (DANIEL KENNEDY) HAVE COME IN CONtact with some remarkable people. I will never forget meeting a D-Day war hero at a conference in Anaheim. This elderly man brought dignity to the uniform. As he told me about that day on the Normandy beach, images from *Saving Private Ryan* raced through my mind. Was the real thing as chaotic and terrifying as the movie? Worse.

"I hit the beach with all of the troops with a very special mission. I was there to give hope to those who were falling. My objective was to transform the fear in those young men's eyes into peace. I was armed only with the Bible. I was an Army chaplain."

My life was changed by that short interaction. How did soldiers cope with threats on their lives? How did they manage anxiety and stress? In the case of that chaplain, his mind was on others, his mission, and God. He survived, and his enduring vision of what he had accomplished helped him cope.

Another person who profoundly affected me was one of my psychology professors, Dr. Beverly Peterson, who once made a statement that I have never forgotten.

All of us need to keep one question in front of us at all times. "What is the difference between me and the person in front of me who is troubled?" The difference is that at a particular moment, in a certain situation, under specific circumstances, I was able to cope and the other person was not.

How a person copes with stress will determine the quality of life he or she enjoys. We have all met people who can let something like getting cut off on the freeway or a delayed flight absolutely ruin their day. You have probably met others who have gone through a divorce, single parenthood, extreme poverty, and still come out saying, "Life is good."

My greatest teachers have been patients with cancer who have honored me with gifts of vulnerability and honesty. Some have shared their deepest fears and greatest joys. All have modeled different coping mechanisms. I have seen people so paralyzed by fear that it was hard to get them out of the car to come in for a consultation. I have seen others try to shoehorn a doctor's appointment into a schedule so hectic they could barely fit us in because they were too busy living to bother.

This chapter deals with the coping mechanisms I have seen to be most effective, as confirmed by clinical studies. One researcher said that people in the oncology field have found cancer patients to be most concerned with:

Coping with the late physical effects of medical treatment; coping with the chronic uncertainty of remission or cure; coping with problems related to intimacy, marriage, and reproduction; and coping with factors related to employment discrimination.[1]

The whole experience of being diagnosed with cancer can go beyond intense all the way to surreal. Other researchers have reported that:

It has been shown that the diagnosis and treatment of cancer may constitute a traumatic event that generates reactions consistent with the symptom profile of posttraumatic stress disorder.[2]

If you are familiar with the term *posttraumatic stress disorder* (PTSD), you have probably heard it in the context of Vietnam veterans who can't cope with the memories and nightmares of war. It is also being diagnosed frequently in people who were sexually molested as children. Likewise, many survivors of the terrorist attacks in New York and Washington will suffer from it.

Cancer is also right up there with such traumatic events. According to Dr. Mari Lloyd-Williams, depression is very common in cancer patients and often goes unreported, unrecognized, and untreated.[3] Patients, family members, and even physicians may all find it difficult to talk about emotional efforts because it opens the door to experiencing pain.

If you have cancer, you may be thinking to yourself, "Yep," or, "I didn't know others felt the way I do." If you don't have cancer, you might believe that cancer patients are preoccupied only with death. But I have found that patients' fear and anxiety are focused more on life and survival. Many questions run through their heads: "Will it be painful and have horrible side effects?" "Will I still be attractive to my husband after the surgery?"

In the previous chapter I suggested that many people even go beyond questions to negative thinking, such as, "Everyone thinks I can't handle my job now that I am taking chemotherapy."

If you or your loved one is faced with cancer, worries such as these are normal. How can you cope with these issues? In the following chart the left side lists several coping strategies that really work, along with several strategies on the right that are not effective or can even be counterproductive.

EFFECTIVE COPING STRATEGIES	INEFFECTIVE COPING STRATEGIES
Problem solving	Denial
Information seeking	Wishful thinking

Effective Coping Strategies	Ineffective Coping Strategies
Fighting spirit	Problem avoidance/escape
Positive reinterpretation	Self-criticism/blame
Self/cognitive restraint	Social withdrawal
Seeking social support	Fatalism
Expressing feelings	Resignation
Using humor	Hopelessness
Seeking religion, faith, prayer	Helplessness
Acceptance	Anger

On the negative side, getting down on yourself and thinking that you caused the cancer leads to depression. It only fuels a vicious cycle of fear breeding fear, anxiety provoking anxiety, and depression duplicating depression.

So how can you cope with the stress of cancer? Bring it out in the open, learn about it, find a good support group, incorporate faith and hope, and develop a healthy way of thinking about it.

Talk to Someone Who Cares!

When people have cancer, they reach out to others, and they talk about it, right? Not really. One research study found that:

> …interventions that increase breast cancer patients' communication with family members lead to reduced patient distress; [conversely] the coping mechanism of escape and silence is common among people who have any type of cancer.[4]

Why do people hide the fact that they have cancer? Many patients don't want to burden others with their problems, or they don't want their children to worry. Others either become nervous and talkative or very still and quiet when they get scared. Others keep quiet because they don't want people to pity them or change the way they act around them.

All these reasons are understandable, but avoiding the subject or keeping quiet increases stress and lowers the quality of life for the patient and everyone around him. Besides, talking about the illness and reaching out for support has been shown to lower psychosocial stress, and it helps facilitate the emotional adjustment.

One of the most important, beautiful things we see at the Oasis of Hope is bonding between patients. We don't suggest to people that they should make friends and support one another, but we have created an environment conducive for that to happen. We don't have our patients wear hospital gowns, and we fill their days with group activities. We serve meals in rooms only when a person is so ill he can't get out of bed. Because everyone is in plain clothes, it is difficult to tell the difference between patients, patient companions, and staff members.

As patients sit down to eat together three times a day, the conversations and support begin. They literally teach each other about the treatment process. They also open up and share their fears and concerns, and they give each other tips on how to cope with those feelings. I have also seen patients pray together for those who are not doing well. And we see a lot of hugging.

This bonding between patients is what I call "friendships for life." Such friendships last for life because they are formed with a common purpose of preserving and extending life for everyone involved.

Information seeking also helps to lower anxiety levels. One of your best resources is the Internet. You can literally educate yourself on a particular type of cancer and the different treatment options. The information is so accessible that many times our patients know as much as our doctors do about their particular illnesses!

We also spend a lot of time teaching our patients about ways to overcome cancer through nutrition, lifestyle, and therapies. And we provide spiritual and emotional resources. In all these ways we constantly support one another and help each other get through difficult times. It is so rewarding to see the transformation of people who are riddled with fear into people who have a peace that passes understanding.

Positive Dialogue

Another effective coping mechanism is self-control/cognitive restraint. Rather than getting carried away by extreme thoughts, we should be realistic about the impact of circumstances. Let me demonstrate this with dialogue very similar to what I have had with numerous patients. You will see how people can let thoughts take them to a place that is not helpful and how getting control of those thoughts can bring stability.

> Patient: *I am dying.*
>
> Therapist: *You are dying right now? Are you having a cardiac arrest, or are you asphyxiating?*
>
> Patient: *No, I don't mean right now. But the doctor says I have only six months to live.*
>
> Therapist: *You have six months to live.*
>
> Patient: *Yes.*
>
> Therapist: *So you are going to live for the next six months.*
>
> Patient: *No, I am dying.*
>
> Therapist: *Did the doctor say you had six months to live or six months to die?*
>
> Patient: *He said to live.*
>
> Therapist: *So you are living.*
>
> Patient: *Yeah, OK, I'm living. But I am going to die in six months.*

Therapist: *You are definitely going to die in six months?*

Patient: *Well, the doctor said that 60 percent of the people who have my diagnosis die within six months.*

Therapist: *So you have a 40 percent probability of living more than six months.*

Patient: *Yeah, but the probability that I will die is greater.*

Therapist: *Actually, you have a 100 percent guarantee that you will die. We all die one day. But are you dying today?*

Patient: *No.*

Therapist: *You have a 100 percent guarantee that you will die in six months?*

Patient: *No, I could survive.*

How can you benefit from this concept? Listen to yourself. If you catch yourself using terms like *always, definitely,* or *everything,* stop yourself and write down what you are saying. Then ask yourself, "Is the thought I am expressing rational?" If it is not, replace it with a rational thought that leaves open the possibility that something good could happen. The chart below includes some examples.

Irrational Statement	Rational Replacement Statement
Bad things always happen to me.	Both bad and good things happen to everyone. That's part of life.
I am definitely going to die in six months.	Doctors say I could die in six months, but whether I have six months or twenty years left, I will live each day to the fullest.

Irrational Statement	Rational Replacement Statement
Everything is my life is terrible.	There are some parts of my life that I am not happy about, but I am going to concentrate on the good things.

Some of the most devastating, irrational thoughts people have when dealing with cancer involve self-blame and self-criticism. I have heard patients say such things as:

- "I must have done something to deserve this."
- "I am weak, and that's why I have cancer."
- "I am not strong enough to overcome cancer."

Not one of those statements is true. They all need to be replaced. Liberating yourself of extreme negative thinking like this is a very important way to undermine cancer's ability to play mind games with you.

Acceptance

The word *acceptance* might be confusing. You shouldn't accept your diagnosis in the sense of rolling over and dying. I mean "acceptance" as the opposite of denial. Acceptance comes when you go through shock, denial, fear, guilt, and anger, then take a breath and say, "OK, I have cancer, and it's a serious disease." That can be followed up with a resolve and a fighting spirit to live through the crisis and get you out to the other side.

Another word that I like better than *acceptance* is *surrender*. One of the best places we can get to is the place of surrender to the Higher Power. When you can say, "My life belongs to God. He had a plan and a purpose for me even before I was born," you are on the way to good emotional health.

Chapter 15

SOUL-SEARCHING TIME: FIND THE WILL TO LIVE

Cancer Beater #15

I F YOU HAVEN'T READ VIKTOR FRANKL'S *MAN'S SEARCH FOR Meaning*, published in 1963, hop on the Internet. You will probably find used copies for less than three dollars, but the message in the book is priceless.

Viktor was a young psychiatrist who was married and expecting a child in Austria at the start of World War II. He was also Jewish. As the rest of the Jewish population was corralled into prison camps, he managed to stay out because he had a Nazi officer as a client. That helped him for a few months, but finally he and his family were split up and sent to different death camps. Viktor had a manuscript that summed up his life's work, which he sewed to the inside of his coat to preserve it. Of course, his strategy failed, and the manuscript was destroyed.

In the midst of horrific suffering and atrocity, Viktor made it his personal mission to reconstruct his manuscript in his mind, piece by piece. Though he was malnourished, abused, stripped of all dignity, dehumanized, and left for dead, he continued to observe the behaviors of prisoners and soldiers. He shares what he witnessed in his book.

His main conclusion was that if man does not find meaning for his life, even meaning in suffering, he will not be able to cope. Later we will see what he discovered about hope.

Viktor had a reason to survive. He hoped to be reunited with his parents, wife, and child. He also hoped to advance his life's work. These reasons gave him the will to survive the death camps. Unfortunately, none of his family did; nonetheless, he went on to make some of the most important contributions to existential psychology of the twentieth century. He died of old age in 1997.

I (Daniel Kennedy) see a lot of parallels with cancer. Cancer can be demoralizing. It threatens to strip away our dignity. It breathes fear into people, and the treatments at times can seem inhumane. It is easy to give in to cancer. I feel sad to say this, but I have met many people who simply lost hope, just as some did in Auschwitz. But others were like Viktor Frankl; they had the will to live, and live they did.

That is how it is with a life-threatening illness. You need to choose not to give in to cancer and not to be intimidated by it. You need to find the will to live.

The Woman Who Did Not Want to Live

Let me tell you about a woman who did not want to live anymore. When she arrived, she had stopped eating and wouldn't talk to anyone. Her husband was desperately trying to save her life, and he would ask all the other patients, every doctor, every nurse, every person on the kitchen staff, and anyone else he could find to go speak to his wife and try to get her to eat and talk.

When he found me, I agreed to go. She wouldn't make eye contact with me. I made small talk, but she wouldn't answer. Finally I told her it was nice to meet her and turned to leave, at which point her fragile hand lifted up and grabbed my own. I turned back to look at her.

"Are you the young man I saw telling another patient about the Book of Ruth?" she asked.

"Yes," I said.

"Would you come by tomorrow and tell me about the Bible?"

The next day I went to see her again. She was in the hospital bed and very weak. Her husband told me that her doctor didn't think she would make it through the day. She was so weak I had to press my ear against her lips to hear her.

"Tell me the plan of salvation," she said.

I told her about how God sent His only Son to reunite us with Him because we had been separated by sin. I told her that all we had to do was receive the gift of Jesus and ask for forgiveness, and we would be given eternal life. Then I asked her if she wanted to receive Christ.

"Son," she said, "I have been a Christian for more than fifty years, but the story of Jesus is so beautiful I just wanted to hear it one more time." She had such peace. I looked at her husband, and he also had peace. A couple of hours later, she went on to be with the Lord.

This was not a story of defeat. This woman had lived a long and fulfilling life, and she was simply ready for the afterlife. She willed herself onward to heaven. It is another example of how important your will is. You can will yourself to live, or you can will yourself to go on to the next life.

What is on the other side of your illness that is worth getting to? I have seen many young mothers determined to survive for their children. Others fight because they want to raise funds for cancer research. Others just want to deny cancer a victory! If you don't have a reason to survive, you probably won't.

Discipline and Determination and Encouragement!

Overcoming cancer also takes a lot of discipline and determination.

At Oasis of Hope we follow up with our patients for five years. Obviously we care about them, but we also have a bigger reason. A number of years ago, we noticed that seven patients who were referred by a doctor back East were all doing well after treatment with us. But seven patients referred by a different doctor all died. The ones who were living continued to receive periodic phone calls from the doctor who had referred them in the first place. He wasn't treating them anymore; he just called to ask them how they were doing and if they were adhering to their home therapies.

We already knew that whether patients would survive after they left the hospital depended to a huge extent on how well they stuck to the therapy and the diet. The typical therapeutic diet includes organic vegetables and fruits, and lots of fresh juice made from fresh produce. All this takes discipline and determination to juice every day and to remember to take all the tablets. And discipline and determination, to an amazing extent, can be reinforced and even "held in place" by someone else who cares enough to offer regular encouragement.

Sadly, many patients without such support abandon treatment because it becomes "too hard." Other times they start feeling better, and they just quit doing the therapy. Please don't do that.

Focus and resiliency are also vital. You must keep focused on the goal to survive no matter what. That can be more difficult than it sounds. A bad day, continued pain, or undesired results from a CT scan can all demoralize you and break your focus. This is where resiliency becomes indispensable. You must will yourself to live no matter what you hear, see, or perceive. And when bad news comes, you must bounce back. When pain comes, you must endure, telling yourself that you can deal with it however intense it gets, and eventually it will go away.

My pastor once told the familiar story of several people who were asked to paint pictures that symbolized peace. Most people painted pictures of sunsets or family picnics, but one man painted a scene of a storm, with the ocean raging and gigantic waves pounding the shore. But he put a huge rock out in the water, all by itself. When asked how his picture represented peace, he said, "Do you see that rock? Even in the presence of a huge and powerful storm, it doesn't move. That's peace."

When a person can have peace no matter what the circumstances, no matter what the status of the disease, cancer has been defeated. It's an internal anchor, a rock, a firm foundation, something inside you that won't be shaken. When you can say, "It is well with my soul," even if the outcome is still unclear, you have become a victor.

Dr. Bernie Siegel's landmark book *Love, Medicine and Miracles* told of many patients who willed themselves to live. His "exceptional cancer patients," as he called them, had a number of traits in common.[1]

- They were generally successful at careers they liked, and they remained employed during their illness or returned to work soon.

- They were receptive and creative but sometimes hostile, having strong egos and a sense of their own adequacy.

- They had a high degree of self-esteem and self-love, and they were rarely docile.

- They retained control of their lives.

- They were intelligent, with a strong sense of reality.

As patients, they were the ones who read or meditated in the waiting room instead of staring forlornly into space. In other words, they were engaged in life. They went out and made things happen. They had a sense of purpose, and they wanted to get back to that as soon as possible. And most important, cancer was just something to deal with, not what defined who they were.

Together, the *desire* and the *reason* to live must precede the *will* to live. You can't have one without the other two. So what is life to you? Why is it worth living? Why is it worth fighting for? What are you going to do in times of pain? How are you going to stick with your treatment plan? If a bad report comes from the doctor, how will you bounce back?

Take the time to answer these questions now. And write your answers down. In so doing you will design a battle plan tough enough to put cancer on the ropes.

Chapter 16

LAUGH ALL THE
WAY TO THE BANK

Cancer Beater #16

W HEN THE MEXICAN REVOLUTION BEGAN, MY (FRANCISCO Contreras) father's family lost everything. As a young boy my father learned hardship firsthand. The loss of comfort and security devastated his family and absolutely broke his father. My grandfather abandoned my grandmother to fend for herself and their five children. He died soon after.

My grandmother became a state teacher. Imagine a teacher in Mexico City in the 1930s! She made barely enough to survive, yet there was a life and vitality to that family that defies explanation.

Somehow, in those years of hardship, my father discovered the healing powers of music, art, humor, and prayer. He learned from experience that these things were medicine to the soul. He learned that life was better when he heard the music and saw the humor. Prayer could get him through a long, hard night, and a painting could inspire him to reach for lofty goals. He worked hard to internalize these lessons.

Music

My father graduated from medical school in 1939 and practiced medicine for almost twenty-five years before opening the Oasis of Hope.

He came to work every day with patient files under one arm, a guitar under the other, and a smile on his face. In the mornings he consulted with patients. In the afternoons he gathered them together to talk about hope, love, and faith. He played songs. He took requests. He invited them to sing along. He offered to put their lyrics to music.

My father studied joke books too, so he could help his patients laugh. He had excellent comic timing, and the jokes were pretty funny, but that wasn't what made the difference. What really made them laugh was the fact that the comedian wore a lab coat and a stethoscope. I never realized the impression that made on people until recently.

A former patient from years ago pulled me aside recently. "You know what I remember about your father?" she asked, tugging at my sleeve. "He made me laugh—really laugh. What do you get when you mix onions and beans?" I shrugged my shoulders. "Tear gas!" She laughed again, and I did too. "Your dad told me that joke!"

My father had a kind word, a song, a joke, and a hug for all his patients. When they were scheduled to leave the hospital, my father would go to their room to sing one last song with them. I have never seen a doctor love his patients as my father did.

My father's legacy lives on through the Oasis of Hope staff today. We continue to love our patients in word, song, and laughter. We understand that we cannot help a patient alter his life if we do not deal with his emotional well-being. Following in our founder's footsteps, we provide activities beyond our counseling program that promote excellent emotional health.

There is no question that music speaks to our hearts in a way mere words cannot. Paul Simon once talked about the song "Only Living Boy." He said he liked the particular chord progression he used to transition to the chorus and that studies revealed it evoked tears. I was fascinated. The fact that music can elicit particular emotions makes it a powerful tool in the hands of a physician.

Clinical research now shows that music can positively influence the respiratory system, the circulatory system, the immune system, and the endocrine system. Indeed, as N'omi Orr once said:

> Military drums play music designed to make your feet take you where your head never would—music is almost as dangerous as gunpowder.[1]

Music can slow your respiratory rate, lower your blood pressure, and bolster your body's defense mechanisms. Music can stimulate the production of endorphins. Couple these effects with the emotional benefits, and maybe you'll agree that more doctors should prescribe music for their patients. Teaching patients to incorporate music into their lives helps them shift their focus off the pain and stress that accompany a battle with cancer.

Art

Want to see something fascinating? Take a man in his forties and show him a box of your kid's Legos. Then say that you need to make a phone call and leave the room for sixty seconds. When you return, he will be playing with the Legos.

There is something about the act of creating something that draws humans as the moon draws water. This is why art therapy is so important. It satisfies the basic human need to be creative. It's also why Oasis is a house of art.

We have original sculptures and paintings all over the hospital, all of which relate to healing and uplifting passages from Scripture. My favorite piece is a bronze sculpture in our prayer center by a famous Mexican artist named Olivia Guzman. She won Mexico's national prize for art in 1988. Looking at this piece, you can see the inspiration and passion she poured into it. It shows the young man who was born blind, with Jesus putting mud on his eyes and sending him to wash in the pool of Siloam.

Making an original work of art can bring happiness and peace.

Creating and talking about art help patients cope with the stress of battling disease. You have heard of catharsis. Putting a brush to a canvas or a pen to paper can be cathartic, and it can really help you deal with your thoughts and feelings about cancer. This is an important way to turn disorganized, irrational thoughts into organized, rational thoughts.

Humor

The first time I listened to Bill Cosby talk about himself and his brother Russell, I laughed so hard I cried. Tears rolled down my face. At one point I had to stop the recording because I couldn't breathe. I actually thought, "If I don't hit the stop button and calm down, I will die!" I pictured my parents walking into my room and finding my body on the floor, hands on my stomach, a smile plastered to my face. Bill Cosby introduced me to the notion that some people are truly gifted at making people laugh.

Do you know there is healing power in laughter? Dr. Norman Cousins knew. When he was diagnosed with a degenerative disease, he checked himself out of the hospital. He then went home and cured himself by adopting a diet of healthy foods, juices, and humor. He didn't get weak medicine either. He didn't settle for the cheap laughs that so many films today embrace. He surrounded himself with comic genius: Chaplin, Laurel and Hardy, Lucy and Desi, and Cosby. He ate, drank, and was merry, and his illness went away.

Don't chalk his success story up to luck, either. He knew what he was doing, about the benefits of good diet and laughter. Laughter helps the body release endorphins, obtain oxygen, and relax tense muscles.

At Oasis, we encourage patients to incorporate humor into their lifestyles. We watch videos featuring gifted comedians. We bring in a laughter therapist. We help patients discover the wide variety of opportunities for laughter in their day-to-day world. We believe the healing power of laughter can help restore a person to a healthy emotional state, and then it can help them maintain that balance.

Prayer

Also, although we will talk more deeply about prayer later on, I want to mention it here because you don't even have to believe in God to benefit from prayer. We pray with all our patients, of every race, culture, religion, and nationality. When people are facing cancer, they become very open. I have prayed with Christians, Buddhists, Muslims, Jews, and even atheists. And I know that no matter where they come from, the prayer will help. Why? Prayer has a natural healing power.

Bringing It All Together

My father and I did not invent music, laughter, art, or prayer. Yet these things make the Oasis of Hope a unique treatment center. Few cancer centers incorporate them into the treatment approach, even though countless clinical trials have confirmed the benefit they can offer patients.

The objective of these powerful therapies is not to create warm, fuzzy feelings but to restore the mind to a balanced emotional state. We have witnessed positive changes in the majority of our patients for more than forty years. That history alone defines who we are at Oasis and who we will continue to be.

But you don't have to come to the Oasis of Hope to get these noetic therapies. (*Noetic* means "relating to or originating in the intellect.") You can implement them in the comfort of your own home.

Chapter 17

DISCOVER THE HIDDEN ROOTS OF ILLNESS

Cancer Beater #17

I (DANIEL KENNEDY) WAS IN MY OFFICE WHEN I GOT AN URGENT call from a patient. "There is a man going from room to room telling patients that they are sick because they are sinful people, and if they don't confess their sins, they will surely die!" I immediately went to look for this intruder, and when I found him, I asked him to leave.

He looked me straight in the eye. "You are the administrator of this hospital! You have authority over what goes on in this place! Because you refuse to confront your patients with their sins, their deaths will be on your head!"

A chill ran down my spine. Was this man crazy, or did he have a point? Do we bring cancer on ourselves because of our sin? What would the Lord have us do?

I began immediately to search for the truth about any possible connection between sin and disease. God's Word is clear that sin and disease do have a direct correlation, but the more powerful message is the promise of the forgiveness He has made available to everyone.

How can we best help people who are ill discover the message of forgiveness and healing? I invite you to explore God's truth in 2 Chronicles 7:14; Isaiah 53:4–5; and James 5:14–16 with me. Through careful study and meditation on these passages, we can see the wonder of God's forgiveness, healing, and salvation come to light, and it is a message that is vital to everyone living today.

Second Chronicles 7:14 reveals to us the promise of God to forgive and heal. Isaiah 53:4–5 explains God's provision of this healing. James 5:14–16 teaches how to apply the promise and provision to our lives. Let us share these truths today so that all may know that they may be forgiven, healed, and saved.

The Promise

If my people, which are called by my name, shall humble themselves, and pray, and seek my face, and turn from their wicked ways; *then* will I hear from heaven, and will forgive their sin, and will heal their land.

—2 CHRONICLES 7:14, KJV, EMPHASIS ADDED

For you to live a fulfilled life, you must be forgiven of your sins and made whole. But what is sin? The Bible clearly expects us to observe the Ten Commandments, but we don't have to murder, rob, or rape to be a sinner. God has literally written the knowledge of good and evil upon our hearts, and though we may condition ourselves not to listen, our consciences generally let us know when something isn't right.

Indeed, I have yet to meet a person who honestly believes he has never done anything wrong. However, most people think the consequences of sin come in eternity. Fewer people understand that sin can have huge consequences during this lifetime. Unpardoned sin brings suffering and death. It leaves each person with the need to be forgiven, healed, and saved.

God made a promise to King Solomon, the third king of Israel, that reveals God's ongoing desire to forgive and to heal everyone. I consider two words in 2 Chronicles 7:14 of significant importance: the words *if* and *then*. These two words clearly indicate that God's promise is conditional—*if* the children of Israel will do something, *then* God will also do something.

Action–reaction

When God created the world, He put many natural laws into place, including the law of gravity. Gravity is a lot like God. You can't see it, but you feel its force. I once had a philosophy teacher who would start every class the same way. He would hold out his car keys and ask, "Is anyone willing to bet that when I release these keys, they won't fall to the ground? Anyone?"

Another thing you probably learned along the way is that for every action there is a reaction. If you stretch a rubber band, it will snap back when you let go. Of course, as a child, I liked to let the band snap my sister's arm, which usually earned me a totally different reaction from my father!

God also put in place a number of spiritual laws. One that Jesus taught us is that we will all reap what we sow. This means you will receive the punishment or reward for the way you live your life. The decisions we make and the actions we take all come with consequences. We see this with every story in Genesis. Adam and Eve did not obey God, and they were cast out of Eden. Thus death entered into the world, childbirth became painful, and it became very hard to make a living. Noah obeyed God when he built the ark, and he and his family were spared. Abraham believed God, and it was credited to him as righteousness. The people of Sodom and Gomorrah refused to repent, and they were destroyed.

Are all sick people sinners?

Now, let's be clear. I am not saying that you have to sin to get sick. You can get sick simply by being in the wrong place at the wrong time. When I was a child, we went to visit some friends who had the chicken pox. My sister got the same thing, even though she hadn't sinned. Conversely, I didn't get sick—but not because I was a saint!

On the other hand, many of us are not sick today because God sends disease in response to our sins but because of the choices we make. If a man with high cholesterol continues to eat fast food, a heart attack will probably follow. God does not need to send the cardiac arrest; the man brings it on himself. The natural laws of physiology, biology, and kinesiology are at work, just as gravity is. If you make unhealthy choices, you will reap disease.

Sometimes God also has His own reasons for allowing an illness to occur. My father learned this lesson some years ago when he suffered from kidney stones. His pain was so great that his doctor sent him to get a CT scan. The scan verified the stones in one kidney, but it also revealed a much greater problem in the other one—cancer. They were able to take out the cancerous kidney before it could spread, but had it not been for the kidney stones, my father might have passed away several years earlier.

To put all this in perspective, Jesus Christ Himself taught that a person who is ill has not necessarily sinned. The ninth chapter of John tells about a man who was born blind. After Jesus restored his sight, the apostles asked Him who had sinned, the man or one of his parents. Jesus told them that this infirmity had been allowed so that the work of God could be manifested in this man.

This is a biblical example of an illness with a purpose. Another example is found in John 11. In the story of Lazarus, Jesus said, "This sickness is not unto death, but for the glory of God, that the Son of God might be glorified thereby" (John 11:4, KJV).

However—and please pay attention because I want you to understand exactly what I'm saying here—many diseases today result directly from sin. Sexually transmitted diseases are the most obvious. If you and your spouse remain faithful to each other, and if neither of you is infected when you marry, it is virtually impossible to get an STD. And I do not agree that "AIDS is God's way of punishing homosexuals," but I do believe that if they would not engage in improper sexual activities, most could avoid the HIV virus.

God keeps His promises

Not only did God promise to forgive and heal, but He also kept His word. Further on in 2 Chronicles you read of the tremendous blessing

God bestowed on Israel, especially on King Solomon. Chapters 8 and 9 tell of the incredible wealth Solomon acquired. Silver became as common as stones.

Unfortunately, all that came to an end when Solomon, who had so greatly honored God in his youth, did the opposite in his later years. First Kings tells us how Solomon gave in to his many wives and began to worship their gods. Because of Solomon's sins, Israel became a divided kingdom and later became enslaved. When Solomon was obedient, God kept His promise of blessing. When Solomon was disobedient, God kept His promise of the curse.

Forgiveness and healing

Have you been sick recently or suffered loneliness, financial difficulties, or anxiety? Do you desire the relief that can come through forgiveness and healing? God wants to give those things to you, but you need to do what was required of the Jews long ago. You must humble yourself, pray, and seek God's face.

Some people tell me that they would like to go to church, but they feel that they need to clean up their act before they could attend. They say they don't feel worthy. The truth is, it takes great humility to go into a place of worship when you know you've been bad. And God wants you to take that step. God wants you to turn from your sinful ways. The original Hebrew text for the word *ways* is *deh'rek*, which means "way, road, distance, or journey." Where has your life's journey taken you?

God will forgive you just as He did in Solomon's time. He may decide to heal you too.

The Provision

Surely he hath borne our griefs, and carried our sorrows: yet we did esteem him stricken, smitten of God, and afflicted. But he was wounded for our transgressions, he was bruised for our iniquities: the chastisement of our peace was upon him; and with his stripes we are healed.

—Isaiah 53:4–5, KJV

Though man brought suffering, disease, and death upon himself, God made a provision by which man may be redeemed. The Holy Spirit insists that you know how you may be forgiven and healed, both for today and forever. God created the world with a perfect balance between Him and His creation. There was no sickness or suffering, and there certainly was no death.

When the original sin was committed, the door to sickness, suffering, and death opened up, and all people then began to experience these things. Because of the sin of each one of us, we face an eternal separation from God, a life and an afterlife full of suffering and affliction without God's intervention. Even if it were possible to be saved by doing good works, no man has ever lived without sinning. No man is worthy to face God on his own merit.

God made a provision by which all can be forgiven, healed, and saved. In Isaiah 53:4–5, the prophet Isaiah told of the future fulfillment of God's provision. It was a message of hope that now has come to pass and is a reality for each of us.

God's relationship with man

The fifty-third chapter of Isaiah reveals the whole wonder of God's love and commitment to mankind. It speaks of the coming of the Lord and what Jesus will do for each of us. Because we have broken the Law, none of us are without sin, and we are unable to redeem ourselves. It took someone who was pure and blameless to make atonement for all, and all of our sins are erased vicariously through the sacrifice of Christ.

Chapter 53 is *the event*! Jesus came to Earth, took all our sin and imperfections upon Himself, and died on our behalf. His resurrection gave us eternal life, and for this the Father has given all riches and glory to Christ, which He will share with those who believe in Him. With the fulfillment of this prophecy, mankind received something more profound than the Law.

We received grace. I thought I understood the magnitude of Christ's sacrifice, but viewing Mel Gibson's *The Passion of the Christ* deepened my appreciation for Jesus's selfless act.

Today, we can be redeemed and healed because Jesus died in our place, and we can live eternally because He was raised from the dead and lives now and forever.

Sometimes when I am counseling people who have cancer, I ask them if they could imagine what it would be like to put everyone's cancer, AIDS, diabetes, leprosy, and every other sickness onto one person. Most patients will tell me that they can hardly hold up under the burden of just one disease. It always hits home when I remind them that Jesus took everyone's illness on Himself.

But the physical diseases were not as crushing as the spiritual offenses.

Forgiven and saved

As I mentioned before, Jesus's sacrifice is the only thing that can redeem you and me. The prophecy in Isaiah 53 does not include the words *forgiveness, pardon, redemption, atonement,* or *salvation,* but the central message of this passage is that Jesus died in our stead precisely to give us all these things. Jesus willingly submitted Himself to a horrible death to save our souls. And God wanted us to be sure we knew we could be saved, and by whom, so He inspired His apostle John to write these scriptures:

> For God so loved the world, that he gave his only begotten Son, that whosoever believeth in him should not perish, but have everlasting life.
>
> —John 3:16, KJV

> These things have I written unto you that believe on the name of the Son of God; that ye may know that ye have eternal life, and that ye may believe on the name of the Son of God.
>
> —1 John 5:13, KJV

In my experience, if there is one thing common to man, it is emotional pain. Many of us are crippled because of it. In counseling situations I often ask, "Who hurt you?" Many times someone else has hurt the individual, but the number one perpetrator is the person himself. We all hurt ourselves greatly by the poor decisions we make.

If you tell a little white lie, it will rebound and hurt you after it hurts others. If you choose drunkenness instead of sobriety, it will hurt you.

What are you doing or thinking that could be causing your suffering? Did you know that when you hurt yourself, you are also offending God?

Whatever pain you have in your life, whatever sickness, whatever sin, it can all be healed if you accept the sacrifice Jesus Christ made for your life.

Deliverance Is Yours

Is any sick among you? let him call for the elders of the church; and let them pray over him, anointing him with oil in the name of the Lord: And the prayer of faith shall save the sick, and the Lord shall raise him up; and if he have committed sins, they shall be forgiven him. Confess your faults one to another, and pray one for another, that ye may be healed. The effectual fervent prayer of a righteous man availeth much.

—James 5:14–16, KJV

You can live a redeemed and healthful life. The Holy Spirit wants you to know of God's promise of forgiveness, healing, and salvation. Embrace His promise, and apply it to your life so that you may be whole, today and forever.

James instructs us to pray for healing, and he adds the promise that God will raise us up. But there is a more profound message of eternal healing that comes through the confession of our sin. A number of significant questions come to mind as we read the fifth chapter of James.

If people are sick, does it mean they have sin in their lives? If people are not healed, is it because of hidden sin in their life, because they do not have enough faith and prayer force, or is it because God was not referring to physical healing in the fifty-third chapter of Isaiah?

What I believe are the answers to these questions will become clear to you as you take a deeper look.

Pray for One Another

I remember walking into the reception area of our hospital and seeing a patient, all connected to his IV solutions, laying his hands on another patient and praying with all his energy, pleading with God to heal the man he was praying for. I knew that the one saying the prayer had cancer and was probably not going to make it. I thought to myself, "God is going to have to answer that prayer. This man is not thinking of himself; he is selflessly putting the need of another in front of his own." I thought of James 5:16, which says the fervent prayer of a righteous man is powerful and effective.

James 5:14 instructs us to ask for prayer when we are sick. We are also to confess any sins we might have. This is the 2 Chronicles 7:14 model applied under the power of the fulfilled prophecy in Isaiah 53:5. James writes that God will hear our prayers, forgive our sins, and raise us up from the sickness. I know that many people hesitate to ask for prayer or resist praying for others when they are sick. I think they are afraid that God might not answer their prayers. My word of encouragement to people who feel this way is not to overthink it; just obey God. If you are sick, get prayed for. If you know someone who is sick, go pray for them.

What If You Are Not Healed?

Do you remember the story I told a few pages ago, of "psycho man" telling my patients that they were ill because they had sin in their lives? Sadly, he's not the only person who has ever felt that way. Common "explanations" for the same belief include:

- The sick person is harboring sin. Sickness came into the world because of sin, and if you sin, it will kill you. OK— James 5:15 reminds us that we should confess our sins even as we pray for healing. There is a sin-disease connection. But let's not forget that Christ Himself demonstrated that not all sickness results from sin. Some has another purpose, as did my father's kidney stones.

- The sick person lacks faith. So many times when Jesus healed people, He talked of their great faith or said, "Your faith has made you well." But some people were healed who had no faith. A father had faith, and his dead daughter was resurrected. Who had the faith? A third party. Likewise, Lazarus's sisters kept mourning him even after Jesus arrived. But then He raised Lazarus up. I don't think it is fair to load up the ill with the accusation that their lack of faith is keeping them sick.

It is hard to accept that sometimes it is not the will of God to heal someone, but that is the true explanation. Each of us will die one day, sooner or later. But God heals us over and over of many different things until it's our time. How often have you been healed of the common cold, the flu, and maybe more serious illnesses?

Since you and I don't know when it will be our time, if you get sick, get prayed for; and if it's not your time, God will raise you up. That is His promise, and God keeps all His promises!

In Summary

If it had not been for sin, none of us would ever face death. There can be no doubt that there is a sin-disease connection. But God loves all of us so much that He wants to forgive each of us and heal us. Second Chronicles 7:14 shows God's desire to forgive and heal, provided that we humble ourselves, seek God's face, and turn from evil.

God thus made a provision by which man may be redeemed. The

prophet Isaiah foretold of the Messiah. Jesus fulfilled the prophecy and suffered greatly to atone for our sin. This is how God intends to heal each of us and save us from eternal suffering.

So if you are physically sick, it does not mean that you are harboring sin! But examine your heart. If you become aware of any sin in your life, confess it, and you will be forgiven. This forgiveness is the healing for spiritual illness, and this is the most significant miracle that can happen in your life. Through Jesus, through His sacrifice and resurrection, you can live eternally. But you must make the choice. Will you humble yourself, seek God with all your heart, repent of your sins, and ask Jesus to be your Lord and Savior?

Chapter 18

TAP INTO THE POWER OF HOPE

Cancer Beater #18

I (DANIEL KENNEDY) WAS THIRTEEN, AND I WAS STANDING IN THE batter's box, trembling. It was my first time up in the Babe Ruth baseball league. The previous year I had played Little League on a miniature field, where every hit looked like a home run and most of us boasted batting averages of .600-plus.

Now I was playing with the big guys on a full-sized field. That night, even as I dreamed of a big hit, a scout from the Los Angeles Dodgers sat in the stands, watching a seasoned pitcher called Moose stare at me. Moose had almost four years and forty pounds on me, plus a fastball clocked at 89 mph.

Talk about intimidation. I kept telling myself to show some courage. I wasn't sure why the coach had picked that moment to throw me in the game. I hadn't played all season because I was the backup second baseman, and the first stringer was the coach's son. But that night, the coach's pride and joy arrived late and got benched. I was the leadoff hitter.

I started negotiating with God, "If you let me get a piece of the ball, I will read my Bible every day."

Zoom, zoom, whooosh! Three strikes and I was out. Moose threw so hard I was paralyzed with fear. I didn't even take a swing. To add insult to injury, three really cute girls had come to the game just to watch me play. If I'd had a tail, I would have tucked it between my legs as I made my way back to the dugout.

Why didn't I swing? The worst that could have happened would be to strike out—but I did that without swinging! Not trying was worse than trying and failing. Besides, even Babe Ruth had more strikeouts than home runs. I didn't even try because I was paralyzed by fear, so scared I became my own worst enemy. Even if Moose had lobbed the ball over the plate, I still would have struck out.

Hope Is the Engine

That's how it often is when someone is diagnosed with cancer. To many, the word *cancer* is synonymous with death—"I know you see me walking around, but I am really dead; it's just a matter of time." Cancer's reputation can destroy a person before he or she even considers the options available.

If you or a loved one has been diagnosed with cancer, don't give up before you try. Together, *you* and *hope* can make an incredible team. Many people survive cancer, so why not you? In fact, if you truly want to get through the crisis, you absolutely *must* develop hope.

Earlier I mentioned Viktor Frankl, a prisoner in Auschwitz during the Holocaust. Two decades after the war, Frankl wrote about how the prisoners became so intimately acquainted with death that they could predict the time a person would die, sometimes within a few minutes.

The key indicator popped up when a prisoner began smoking his cigarettes. In the prison camps, cigarettes were like money. People didn't smoke them anymore than you would light up a twenty dollar bill. If a person began to smoke, it meant that he'd given up. Frankl and his fellow prisoners recognized a direct correlation: the absence of hope brought the onset of death.

Hope is to life what an engine is to a car. It *drives* you; it moves you toward a goal. In Spanish, the word for "hope" is *esperanza*, which comes from the verb *esperar*, meaning "to wait, to expect." Thus hope also involves waiting, with desire and reasonable confidence, for circumstances to change so your expectations can be met.

"Most people," Will Rogers said, "are about as happy as they make up their minds to be." In other words, you can change, adapt, or reframe your perceptions and view your world from whatever perspective you wish.

However, if your mind is still reluctant to embrace hope, let me remind you that, as John Johnson once said, "Men and women are limited not by the place of their birth, nor by the color of their skin, but by the size of their hope." Proverbs 13:12 says, "Hope deferred makes the heart sick, but a longing fulfilled is a tree of life" (NIV). Do not let cancer devastate you because you're low on hope.

Never a Hopeless Endeavor

Never forget that cancer is a *condition*, but hope is an *attitude*—a positive attitude that will motivate you to work *with enthusiasm* toward success. I emphasize the word *enthusiasm* because it stems from two Greek words—*en*, which means "in," and *theos*, which means "God." When you do things with enthusiasm, you do them as if you were doing them for God.

Now, *success* is quite subjective because it can mean one thing to you and a different thing to someone else, but I like what Winston Churchill said: "Success is going from failure to failure without loss of enthusiasm." He lost many battles, but he won the war because he never lost hope.

Perhaps the most important message of this book is that fighting cancer need never be a hopeless endeavor.

Lift Up Your Eyes

I believe that faith correlates to the "lift up mine eyes" portion of Scripture below:

> I will lift up mine eyes unto the hills, from whence cometh my help.
> —PSALM 121:1, KJV

Several top universities, including Duke, have done studies on faith, one of which concluded that patients who have religious faith recover from illness more quickly than those who have none.[1] Another concluded that those who have faith were able to get off medication faster and suffer less complications.[2]

From my own experience I know that patients who believe they will overcome cancer do so more often than those who feel uncertain. And people who believe they will die usually do.

How does faith work? On the physical level, what we believe and how we think about things can generate peace and security or just the opposite.

Faith on the Physical Level

When you have peace within, your body relaxes. This takes the stress off your immune system and increases the production of endorphins. If you truly believe you will get well, you will lower your stress and allow your body to concentrate on doing its physical best to fight disease.

Conversely, emotional disturbance takes a physical toll. We begin to suffer headaches, upset stomachs, backaches, and depressed immune systems. In other words, if you truly believe you will not get well, you will add stress to your body and compromise your immune system.

Faith is also important with respect to your treatment choices. If you don't have faith in your physician and the treatment he is prescribing, at the very least it will be less effective than it could be. But if you really believe your treatment will help you, it probably will, even if it is chemotherapy.

Given all that, and since there's no "neutral" position, from a physical perspective alone it makes far more sense to believe something positive rather than something negative.

Dr. Bernie Siegel encourages his patients who opt for radiation and chemotherapy to visualize the treatments working against the cancer and not producing negative side effects. They draw pictures of the positive work the therapy is doing. Dr. Siegel has documented how their positive attitudes toward cancer and their treatment choice truly generate better outcomes than the outcomes other cancer patients have.

Faith on the Spiritual Level

Faith, on the spiritual level, is an important ingredient in many healings documented in the Bible. Remember the faith of the Canaanite woman who refused to give up until Christ healed her daughter (Matt. 15:22–28)? If this was our only reference, it might be easy to conclude that without that kind of faith healing cannot come. But that is not necessarily true.

Remember the four friends who brought a paralytic to Christ? They could not reach Him because of the crowd, so they opened a hole in the roof of the house Christ was in and lowered the man and his bed. The Bible records that when Christ saw the faith of the man's friends, He forgave the man's sins and healed him (Mark 2:2–12). The patient was healed, yet he was not the one whose faith Jesus commended.

Jesus was also impressed with the faith of the centurion who asked Him to heal his servant, who was at the centurion's home. Jesus immediately wanted to go to the servant, but the centurion told Him that wasn't necessary, that Jesus just needed to say the word and it would be done (Matt. 8:5–10). The centurion's faith got it done.

Finally, remember the woman who had the disease in her blood (Mark 5:25–34)? She had *powerful* faith in her treatment choice! She literally believed that if she could just touch the hem of His garment, she would be healed—and she was!

How did people like these develop their faith? To some extent, in addition to what miracles God could have wrought strictly within their hearts, they might actually have seen God work "in the flesh." In the present age, one of the most effective ways is to simply ask God to increase our faith and keep asking until He does.

But you can also do some things by simply using the mental tools God gave you. Several years ago I met Dr. John Huffman, a psychologist who has developed a unique counseling approach called pneumiatrics.

Pneuma means "air" or "spirit," and *iatria* means "physician" or "therapy." So *pneumiatrics* means "spirit therapy," in which several staff members at Oasis of Hope (including me!) have since been trained and certified by Dr. Huffman himself.

I watched Dr. Huffman obtain immediate results working with patients who had previously been bounced around to twenty different psychiatric hospitals without being helped. Later on, when he came to Oasis of Hope, he helped us develop a list from the Bible on how to build faith. Here it is:

- Ask God to give you more faith.

- Read God's promises.

- Write them out.

- Say them aloud in a strong voice.

- Do what is written in the Bible.

- Spend time with people of great faith.

- Ask others to believe along with you, adding their faith to yours and yours to theirs.

- Listen to the testimonies of others whose faith is strong.

- Ask Jesus to have faith *for* you.

If you do these things actively, your faith will increase, and eventually you can make the important transition from *having faith* to *trusting God so completely* that your faith becomes a total surrender to His sovereignty.

Consider the story of Shadrach, Meshach, and Abednego.

These were three Jewish young men who had been abducted from Jerusalem when it fell. They were living in Babylon when the king decreed that all should bow down and worship a golden image. Shadrach, Meshach, and Abednego would not do it. They would not violate God's first commandment by worshiping anyone or anything but Him.

The consequence of breaking the Babylonian king's decree was death in a fiery furnace. Yet when the king gave the young men one last opportunity to change their minds and bow down to the false image, here's how they responded:

> Shadrach, Meshach and Abednego replied to the king, "O Nebuchadnezzar, we do not need to defend ourselves before you in this matter. If we are thrown into the blazing furnace, the God we serve is able to save us from it, and he will rescue us from your hand, O king. But even if he does not, we want you to know, O king, that we will not serve your gods or worship the image of gold you have set up."
>
> —DANIEL 3:16–18, NIV

In other words, these young men had so much faith in God they were willing to bet their lives on it. And God saved them in a miraculous way.

Negative Faith—Again!

Finally, let's address negative faith, usually called doubt. Doubt comes when your faith in God's ability to help is weaker than your fear of a threat. Christ taught that we should not be anxious or fearful. But with so many threats to our health—cancer, drive-by shootings, car accidents, and now even acts of terrorism—how can we avoid being fearful? The answer is that our faith must be rooted in our fear of the Lord.

When you fear God as He intended, meaning that you know and respect Him and have a relationship with Him, you also know that He has the power and desire to protect you. Any fear other than the fear of God can be categorized as the fear of man and the doubt of God, which can lead to various forms of idolatry.

That is why I encourage you to focus on God and not fear cancer. Don't bow down to cancer. Stand up to it, and let it know that the Lord your God will give you victory over it.

Two psalms in particular have become anchors for patients at the Oasis of Hope. I encourage you to read Psalms 23 and 91 on a daily basis, especially if the fear of cancer seems to be getting the best of you.

Fear of cancer is gloriously undermined by faith in God.

Chapter 19

DON'T OVERLOOK
PRAYER THERAPY

Cancer Beater #19

HE'S LOST A LOT OF BLOOD," THE DOCTOR TOLD THE parents. Johnny was riding his motorcycle when a car turned left in front of him. The crash tore off one of his legs. After six hours of surgery, the doctors were able to save the other leg, but Johnny had lost so much blood he was still in serious trouble. "We've done everything that's medically possible. All we can do now is pray," the doctor said.

A Last Desperate Act?

Prayer is often considered the desperate act of the defeated, a last resort. Yet if more doctors faced the facts about prayer as a healing agent, they would embrace it as the first line of defense.

Vast quantities of research documenting the therapeutic benefits of prayer have been around for a long time. If doctors need to be convinced that prayer has medicinal value, they need only consult their industry's journals. The scientific data derived from hundreds of clinical trials performed in reputable universities and hospitals have already been published.

For example, in July 1988, the *Southern Medical Journal* published Dr. Randolph C. Byrd's study "Positive Therapeutic Effects of Intercessory

Prayer in a Coronary Care Unit Population." Perhaps no other clinical trial on prayer has been surrounded by so much attention.

Dr. Byrd, a resident cardiologist, took 393 patients from the San Francisco General Hospital Coronary Care Unit and put their names into a computer. The computer randomly divided the patients into two groups. One group, the "prayer group," was prayed for by a home group of Christians. The patients in the control group did not receive prayer. This double-blind study (called that when neither patients nor physicians are aware of which patients are receiving the treatment—in this case, prayer—and which are not) adhered to the same stringent guidelines that all pharmaceutical studies have to abide by to be considered valid.

The results showed that prayer was a significant therapeutic agent. Not one patient from the prayer group required an artificial airway and ventilator, whereas twelve from the control group did. In addition, prayer group patients were five times less likely to require antibiotics and three times less likely to develop complications than their control group counterparts.[1] Trust me—Dr. Byrd's study raised some eyebrows within the medical community!

Several similar studies have been conducted since. The most recent of these was conducted at Duke University by cardiologist Mitch Krucoff, MD. He launched a pilot study of 150 angioplasty patients. The preliminary results suggested that patients who received prayer in addition to conventional medical treatment experienced a 50 percent to 100 percent better recovery rate than those patients who did not.[2]

In September 1977, the prestigious *New England Journal of Medicine* published a study comparing two groups of patients who had been recommended for bypass surgery. One group chose to forgo the surgery and pray instead. The two-year survival rate of the patients who underwent the surgery was 86 percent. The two-year survival rate of the patients who chose prayer instead was an astounding 87 percent.[3]

While pharmaceutical companies have full-time sales reps and five-inch-thick books to keep physicians apprised of the prescription drugs at their disposal, is there anyone telling doctors about the therapeutic value of prayer?

The answer used to be no, but times are changing. Many medical schools have added the study of prayer to their curriculum, along with other topics that examine the relationships among body, mind, and spirit. This trend is due, in part, to public demand. Only 5 percent of doctors now say they should pray with their patients, but national surveys consistently show nearly 80 percent of patients want their physician to consider their spiritual needs.

Prayer has therapeutic value. Scientists and skeptics may continue trying to explain it away if they are unwilling to embrace the existence of the loving Creator, but those who believe in the Almighty recognize a great deal of healing potential in prayer. I do not believe in a specific formula that will coerce God into action. However, I know that Scripture does specify what we are to do.

> Is any one of you sick? He should call the elders of the church to pray over him and anoint him with oil in the name of the Lord. And the prayer offered in faith will make the sick person well; the Lord will raise him up. If he has sinned, he will be forgiven. Therefore confess your sins to each other and pray for each other so that you may be healed. The prayer of a righteous man is powerful and effective.
>
> —James 5:14–16, NIV

Prayer represents a powerful therapeutic force. The Bible says so, and science continues to confirm that truth. God has always healed through prayer. I have personally witnessed spontaneous remissions as well as slow, steady improvement as a result of prayer. I have also seen how prayer can bring a person into peaceful preparation for the next life. I not only condone the use of prayer at the Oasis of Hope, but I am also thrilled to prescribe it to all of our patients. Prayer is effective, nontoxic, and free. I know of no other therapy that has so many positive aspects and is totally free of negative side effects.

Does Prayer *Always* Work?

More than 350 research papers have been published in scientific journals about the power of prayer. Interestingly enough, about half "prove" that it works, and the other half "prove" that it doesn't.

So, is God only 50 percent effective? Testing God's healing capabilities, if you want to look at it that way, has always struck me as irreverent to say the least. But even in Dr. Byrd's study, "God's success rate" was not close to 50 percent. Some may say that the people praying were not "born again" or "Spirit filled." But no matter who prays, the success rate is never 100 percent.

It is as unreasonable to expect that God will heal everyone as it is to expect that God will answer everyone's prayers with a yes. When patients can accept this, they rise to a new level of peace.

Let's imagine for a moment that God answered every prayer. What would happen? For one thing, if God answered every prayer for healing, the world would be vastly overpopulated by now. And think about how chaotic everything would be. Someone would be praying fervently for rain for his garden while his next-door neighbor would be praying for sunshine. Each is asking God to be with him in his corner of a boxing match. What would happen?

It would be impossible for God to be more than 50 percent effective, even if He were unwise enough to get into such a mess. Which, of course, He isn't.

An Unpredictable God?

At Oasis of Hope Hospital, we maintain a constant prayer chain. When a child is among our patients, our staff suffers more emotionally than at any other time. Even other patients start saying things such as, "I would rather God take me than that child." Then when a child dies, we are perplexed. We prayed over the child, anointed the child with oil, and were all in agreement for the healing, but the child still passed away. Why?

Some may be critical of a God who seems so unpredictable, who often seems to make no finite sense. But we see only in part while God sees the whole. He has a master plan, and what must come to pass will come to pass.

Our finite minds are incapable of grasping God, which I believe is by design. If we were able to understand God and His ways, we would rely on that understanding. An easy formula would lead to manipulation of God's power to meet our capricious needs. Then, instead of depending on God, we would depend on our own ability to master the formula.

God does not want that. He wants us to be utterly dependent on Him.

I believe that prayer is powerful and vital. It is one of the most effective tools you have to undermine cancer. But there is something more valuable than a physical cure. It is the certainty of your eternal future. This is why I am open with patients about my belief in Jesus Christ. The advantage Christians have is eternal. Some people may pray for healing and be healed. We can pray for healing, and if we are healed, great! If not, we still have eternal life with Christ.

Prayer Mission

In 1995, I (Daniel Kennedy) sat down with my family to a lovely Thanksgiving dinner. Before we blessed the meal, my father said, "I have something I need to share with the family. I don't know quite how to say this, but I have been diagnosed with cancer."

Wow, what a blow to all of us. I had never seen an entire turkey feast go to waste, but none of us had any appetite. However, I had already been working with cancer patients for a few years, so I thought, "Now it is time to practice what I preach!"

I asked my father if I could pray for him. "Lord," I said when he agreed, "if it is Your plan to take my dad home to be with You, I won't try to stop You, because I submit to Your will. But now that I have said that, let me tell You what is really on my heart. You already have my mother up there in heaven. I don't have any children yet, but when I do,

I want them to know their grandpa. So, please heal my father."

A few days later, I was praying in my office. I had told God how important it was for patients to receive emotional and spiritual support but that Oasis of Hope is only big enough to treat about six hundred patients per year. And that is hardly anyone considering the millions of people living with cancer. I asked God what could be done to touch the lives of people who would never come to Oasis. The answer that came to me was "prayer."

Prayer was the answer, because prayer is effective at a distance. I called Dr. Contreras and told him, "You know what we are going to do? We are going to initiate a worldwide day of prayer for people who have cancer."

Dr. Contreras's first response was, "If you want to communicate this to the world, it is going to take a lot of money. I will give you $50,000 to help get this off the ground."

Let me tell you, I spent all of that money lightning fast. You can't even send a postcard to all of the churches in America for fifty grand! That was when I discovered the Internet. This tool helped us really bring the message to the world.

We started the worldwide Cancer Prayer Day with the help of Robert A. Schuller on June 5, 1998. To date, we have received tens of thousands of prayer requests through www.cancerprayerday.org from more than one hundred countries. These include places like Slovakia, Denmark, Iceland, Israel, Kuwait, Egypt, Nigeria, South Africa, Australia, Hong Kong, Singapore, Taiwan, Korea, Japan, Colombia, Venezuela, Mexico, and many more. By the way, if you want Dr. Contreras to pray for you, go to the same Internet site and click the Prayer Request button. We receive each request and hand-write the names into a book to pray over.

What started out as a prayer day has become a mission. In the last few years, Dr. Contreras and I have traveled to every continent except Antarctica, carrying the prayer request book to meet with spiritual leaders for prayer. That book holds thousands of names and weighs more than twenty pounds. That might not sound like much, but when I carried it from San Diego, California, to the prayer mountain in Seoul, Korea, and then to Tokyo, Japan, let me tell you, I was feeling it!

Probably the most important thing for someone who has cancer is to know that others care. Praying for a person lets them know precisely that.

A person once asked me, "If God heals everyone of cancer, won't that put you out of business?" I said yes, and that is my biggest dream. I would love to close the hospital because the world was free of cancer! I think I would make a good greeter at Wal-Mart.

Another person asked, "If God heals the world of cancer, will you continue with the Cancer Prayer Day?" My response was, "Absolutely!" I would make sure to pray every day to thank God for ridding this world of such a terrible disease.

How can a prayer be made more effective? The answer is found throughout Scripture and reflected in the next chapter.

On October 21, 1997, a precious little girl named Estela was born. This little angelic being was the first child to be born to my wife, Veronica, and me. To see her little fingers and hear her tiny voice cry out, "I'm here, please hold me," was one of the most intense experiences my wife and I ever shared together. Shortly after Estela's arrival, my father walked into the hospital room and picked up his first granddaughter. As I was watching him hold her, instantly the prayer I had prayed two years earlier came to my mind. I started to cry tears of joy. God had answered my prayer and healed my dad of cancer so that my children would have a grandfather!

Chapter 20

ACCESS YOUR HEAVENLY RESOURCES

Cancer Beater #20

EVEN THE MOST PRIMITIVE CULTURES THROUGHOUT HISTORY have been familiar with various procedures they believed would help heal the sick. Whether many of those methods were actually effective is an open question, but little by little, many people began to note that the human body definitely does respond to certain things in predictable ways. They observed that certain foods produced specific effects. So began the art of medicine.

The Greeks learned to distinguish the symptoms of certain diseases, observing that specific infirmities were subject to natural laws and generally responded to specific remedies. In our day, we ratify the efficacy of many such cures when we use so-called "natural" medicines. The body cries out for what it needs. Thus, when we have the flu, our bodies call for herbal teas, chicken soup, and rest. Less money and fewer lives would be lost if we would just listen!

Instinct is one of the mechanisms God has given us for the preservation of our health. We might also call it organic wisdom. Unfortunately, modern science and its practitioners—especially medical doctors—have gradually separated us from these instincts. But that's not all medical science has done. It has also encouraged us to disregard the emotional impact and the spiritual needs that illness brings with it.

Many modern Christian believers, who accept spiritual guidance in many other aspects of their lives, are somehow terrified of germs. Though many believe in the supernatural power of God, when it comes to health they put their trust in antibiotics and medical treatments. In the past one hundred years especially, we have lost touch with our Creator and learned to put more and more of our trust in science. It pains me (Dr. Contreras) to admit this, but medical doctors have much to do with the prevailing attitude of today, which suggests that all things must be susceptible to scientific proof or they can't be true.

Never mind that down through recent centuries we've seen regular revolutions in scientific thinking on almost every subject, which suggests that no matter how much we think we've learned, much of today's scientific truth could be tomorrow's folly.

However, more important in the here and now, an overreliance on science as the prime authority can destroy the faith of many cancer patients who might otherwise be more willing to depend on God.

God: Creator or Created?

Philosophy suggests that belief in God is a weakness. We need God so much that we invent Him or create Him. The agnostics say it is easier for a person to believe in God or to become very religious when overcome by illness because we want a miracle. But believers affirm that God is our Creator and is able to do what man can't.

In times of pain, we can draw near to seek His grace and His help. "God is our refuge and strength, a very present help in trouble" (Ps. 46:1, KJV). Those who accept the existence of a divine Creator thus have access to spiritual blessing. Clearly, those who genuinely love God and sustain a close relationship with Him can confront disease with greater strength. As we have shown in previous chapters, we set certain intrinsic biochemical mechanisms in motion by our emotional and spiritual states.

Neither philosophy nor science denies this. The only question those disciplines cannot answer is how those mechanisms can sometimes be stood on their heads when healings take place that have no scientific explanations.

Love, Hope, and Optimism

Sadly, that we are children of an almighty God who actually cares about our problems is still considered by many people to be a mythical concept. To them, God is not a being, much less a "person" of action. Yet Christ Himself said:

> Which of you fathers, if your son asks for a fish, will give him a snake instead? Or if he asks for an egg, will give him a scorpion? If you then, though you are evil, know how to give good gifts to your children, how much more will your Father in heaven give the Holy Spirit to those who ask him!
>
> —Luke 11:11–13, niv

If science convinces you that this is unreasonable, you cannot take advantage of the benefits faith provides. On the other hand, if you embrace the offer instead and put your trust in God, your perceptions about life and its problems begins to shift. The actions of God are often suffocated and strangled because we don't acknowledge what we are in Christ. Romans 8:37 says, "In all these things we are more than conquerors through him that loved us" (kjv).

So how to bring all this together?

Love

Jack Medoli and Yuri Goldbert have done a most revealing work in Israel. These two researchers studied ten thousand men with high-risk conditions, such as angina pectoris, anxiety, high cholesterol, and irregular heartbeat. All had one or more classic preconditions for a fatal cardiovascular condition.

Medoli and Goldbert then determined through psychological tests which of the men would develop a heart attack and which would not.

After all was said and done, the ones who had the highest incidence of heart attacks were the ones who answered no to one seemingly innocuous question: "Does your wife show you love?"[1]

Insurance companies have long known that men who are sent off in the morning with kisses from their wives are better clients because they have fewer car accidents. They will also live, on the average, five years longer.[2] If insurance companies were not in the business of evaluating risk to increase their revenue, I wouldn't believe it, either, but there it is, simple and scientific!

Ironically, these revolutionary findings of the twentieth century were well known centuries ago by the Hebrew people. "Rejoice with the wife of thy youth" (Prov. 5:18, KJV). "He who finds a wife finds a good thing" (Prov. 18:22, NAS).

Although love research is still in its infancy, studies are beginning to confirm its positive effects. The Meneger Foundation found that people who are in love have lower levels of lactic acid in their bloodstreams, which causes them to feel less tired. They also have higher levels of endorphins, which cause them to feel more euphoric and less sensitive to pain. Likewise, their white corpuscles respond better to infection, and they catch fewer colds.[3]

In 1982, Harvard psychologists David McClelland and Carol Kirshnit discovered that even films about love increase human levels of immunoglobulin-A in saliva, the first line of defense against colds and other viral diseases.[4] Although this immunological improvement typically lasted less than an hour, it could have been prolonged by having the subjects think about moments in their lives when someone loved them. If we love we are happy, and those around us who love us make up a part of our positive world. And they don't wear down our defenses.

Two Stories

A young woman, nineteen years old, came in to see me. Her doctors had given up hope and diagnosed her with cancer of the small intestine. A course of chemotherapy offered no positive results. Under these conditions, her prognosis was death within three to six months.

This girl was a member of her country's horseback riding team, which in eight months would participate in the Olympic games in Montreal. She said she had come to me because she did not accept the prognosis of her doctors and that under no circumstances would she stay out of the competition.

She began her treatment with a lot of faith and discipline. The results were indeed amazing. In all sincerity, our results with patients with this type of tumor are usually not encouraging, but the determination and tenacity of this girl stimulated her defenses so powerfully that they destroyed her tumor.

However, in reality the treatment only served as an emotional reinforcement. All she needed was someone to give her hope, someone who would show interest and love. Now several years later, this patient is still alive and healthy.

On the other side of the coin, a woman with breast cancer came to us after having been treated surgically. Surgeons had removed her left breast. Her cancer had been complicated by metastasis in the bones and lungs. Conventional therapies had failed, and her doctors had sent her home to die. At the start of our treatment, we could faintly see signs of her former beauty, even though she looked as though she had been in a concentration camp, skeletal and bald. All of this resulted from an aggressive, unsuccessful treatment with chemotherapy.

Little by little she began to improve. Her hair grew back, she gained weight, and the beauty of her face began to reappear. In six months she was a new person. Although an aggressive surgery had dealt her a powerful blow, she overcame it.

But then her husband asked her for a divorce. Under any circumstances this would be a devastating event, but here it was made worse because she interpreted it as a rejection of her disfigured body. Within three weeks she experienced an explosion of tumors.

Although she came back to see me, she confessed that the loss of her husband's love represented the worst kind of rejection and that life had lost all meaning. No human power could change her perspective. Her immune system gave up, and the tumors took advantage of the open doors and killed her.

Love is so important and powerful that Christ summarized six commandments into one, the Golden Rule: "Love your neighbor as you love yourself." Yes! John Lennon was right when he sang that the only thing we need is love. But why is there so little of it?

On the other hand, my brother-in-law, an independent minister, believes that there are so many problems in our world precisely because we love our neighbors as we love ourselves! That sounds like a contradictory perspective, but let's examine how we love ourselves. We love junk food, alcoholic beverages, and smoking. Love is never having to exercise. Our love affair with quarreling, fighting, and hating is at an all-time high. Your neighbor certainly doesn't need this kind of love.

Spiritual Ties

Essentially we are designed to be unified creatures, but the pace of modern life doesn't leave us much room to cultivate whole and balanced lives, unifying body, mind, and spirit. We cannot be divided and yet remain healthy. Those who give exclusive importance to the body but neglect the mind and the spirit fail to practice adequate medicine.

Many famous psychologists—Jung, for example—recommend the cultivating of the spirit to help preserve health. By the word *spirit*, some do not refer precisely to the relationship of the human being to God, but rather to a relationship to beauty through art. Yet I have found through my medical practice that the cultivation of the spirit can really only be understood as the relationship of a man or a woman with God.

The spirit is that part of our being that enables us to communicate with God, who is Himself a spirit. It is what enables hopeless human beings to recover the essence of life in a supernatural way, to discover life as they have never experienced it before.

The patients who throw in the towel almost always do so because of the negative attitudes of their doctors, demonstrated when they say, "There is nothing more to do." But our hearts tell us that hope dies last. In my experience there is much dignity in the struggle, in fighting the invincible foe. Even when hope fails, you earn a feeling of satisfaction from having given the enemy a tough fight. Life, to a great degree, is at our disposal. We have control over our decision to fight or fold. We can't change the past, but we can influence the present and the future by wearing the armor of hope.

Every person who has spiritual ties, regardless of their chosen religion, lives longer and better. But to repeat what I consider the most important point here, our great advantage is that *Christianity* is *founded on love.* "For God so loved the world that he gave his only begotten Son, that whosoever believeth in him should not perish, but have everlasting life" (John 3:16, KJV). This manifestation of God's love to mankind is what enables us to love ourselves and others. It also is the foundation of our hope that whatever we do is not in vain, that we are going to a special eternal place where there will be no more sorrow or pain.

Resources: Scarcity vs. Abundance

To see the human being as a trinity—body, mind, and spirit—and to treat him as such in the practice of medicine is something I learned from my father. When I chat with my patients, I make sure they leave with literal *hope* that can help them confront their condition. As I broach the subject of stress, which is very common, I define it as a deficit of resources needed to resolve a problem. This is a simple definition but adequate. If you have enough money to pay the rent, there is no stress; but anxiety reigns when you hear the footsteps of the landlord and you have to give him an excuse. To tie all this in with music and laughter, think of the scene with Benoit (the landlord) in the first act of *La Bohème,* if you're familiar with that opera!

Success against any adversity requires that you recognize and face the obstacles first. But beyond that, you have to use the resources you have at hand in a positive, optimistic way. It is an illusion to hope for a life without problems, but it's entirely realistic to ask God for help. At Oasis of Hope Hospital, patients get bodily resources, but they are also presented with the opportunity to receive Christ as their Savior, because He is the inexhaustible fountain of resources.

This is why patients with strong spiritual ties to God can better face disease. They can deal with the initial rage, frustration, and despair that all people experience when they find out they are suffering from a serious disease. They trust in God, and they have hope. They maintain a positive spiritual attitude because they fortify themselves with prayer and by reading His Word. The patient who knows he is saved through the provision of Christ does not fear death, because he knows where he is going.

Many others cast aside these concepts as simplistic, but they forget that all human beings in every culture and religion know intuitively that we are spiritually eternal. As a doctor, I am concerned about giving my patients good quality for their fleeting physical life, but shouldn't I be concerned about their eternal life as well?

EPILOGUE

THIS IS THE FOURTH BOOK THAT I (FRANCISCO CONTRERAS) HAVE written specifically about cancer. My first book on the subject was called *The Hope of Living Cancer Free*, which is still one of my favorites because of all the people who have told me how it lifted their spirits.

Daniel Kennedy and I wrote another book in 2004, called *Dismantling Cancer*. But the book that might have been the most controversial was called *The Coming Cancer Cure*. That title provoked many reactions because the title makes it seem that I, as the author, was promising a cure. Let me clarify that and also reinforce the last few chapters of *this* book.

I believe with all my heart that the cure to cancer is coming. I believe that Jesus is coming too. I am not sure if the cure to cancer will come first or if the return of Jesus Christ will make it unnecessary. There are still many things we don't know about cancer. Because of its ability to mutate, it remains mostly a mystery. Even though we know that everything about cancer can be pinpointed at the DNA level, we do not yet know how to stop it.

Each portion of this book was written to explain a different aspect of cancer and to provide specific actions you can take to come against it. We spent a lot of words on diet and lifestyle, for obvious reasons. You can lower your cancer mortality risk by 60 percent just by adapting healthy lifestyle changes!

When I am interviewed, people sometimes ask me, "What can I do to prevent cancer? And don't talk to me about diet and lifestyle!" They would rather pop a pill than give up the way they eat and live. So sad.

We also told you about specific nutrients and foods that can help reprogram abnormal cells and convert them back to healthy cells. We addressed the failings and successes of conventional and alternative therapies. (Don't forget to dig into those endnotes when you want more information on a topic.)

We also spoke at length about the importance of building your emotional health and of finding the will to live.

Finally, we talked about spiritual issues. Spiritual victory over cancer is the most important for everyone because it has eternal consequences.

I believe that all of these things are part of the solution and can really be of help. Much still needs to be learned. Meanwhile, you will drastically improve your prognosis and quality of life if you take all the information we've presented here and begin to live it.

Unless Jesus returns to gather His children to Himself while we live, we're all eventually going to experience a physical death. We hope it is not cancer that does this, but it is possible. We have written this book to help you stand your ground and fight this enemy called cancer. Yet we also wish you to know the peace that passes understanding while you still live. When Jesus Christ reigns in your heart, you can face cancer—and even the thought of death—with the quiet assurance that in Him you will find your final healing.

Our thoughts and prayers are with you as you or a loved one faces this challenge. Our desire is to help people help their doctors defeat cancer. We would also appreciate hearing from you on how this information helped you. Send an e-mail to us at health@oasisofhope.com.

May you continue to receive all the blessings God has for you.

Appendix

THE OASIS OF HOPE
CANCER TREATMENT CENTERS

F
RANCISCO CONTRERAS'S FATHER, DR. ERNESTO CONTRERAS Sr., was at least forty years ahead of his time when he opened Oasis of Hope in 1963. His purpose was to minister to the needs of the whole person—body, mind, and spirit.

However, Dr. Contreras never abandoned conventional medicine—on the contrary, he pioneered it! After completing a fellowship in pediatric pathology at Boston Children's Hospital at Harvard, he became the very first pathologist in northwestern Mexico. He also served hospitals in San Diego, California, in the late 1950s.

Dr. Ernesto Contreras had only one objection to the traditional medicine he was schooled in. Its primary objective was to eradicate disease. Often this led to very aggressive therapies that brought more harm to the patient than the disease. He was also astounded at the number of unnecessary surgeries that were being performed and the number of misdiagnoses that were taking place.

Gradually he concluded that many of these errors were due to the traditional separation doctors maintained from their patients. Doctors were instructed in medical school to avoid personal relationships with patients to protect and maintain their own objectivity. But Dr. Contreras felt that the only way to identify the true needs of his patients was to get to know everything about them.

Thus Dr. Contreras changed his objective from eradicating disease to providing physical, emotional, and spiritual resources according to the needs of the individual, thus bringing his patients back into balance and enabling their bodies to heal themselves. He often found that what a patient needed was not a drug but vitamins or minerals. He also noted that a depressed person often responded better to treatment if he first had sessions of laughter therapy and counseling.

Music, laughter, and prayer, combined with a nutrition program and natural therapies, eventually gained Oasis of Hope an undeserved reputation as an "alternative" hospital. That was never the goal, and this is not an accurate perception. Instead, Oasis of Hope provides *integrative medicine*, which is, instead, a proven combination of conventional and alternative medicine. Truly, what particular treatment is used in any particular instance is not the important consideration. What matters much more is *why, when, how, and in combination with what* a specific treatment is used.

For many years now, medical decisions made by the doctors at Oasis of Hope have been based on the foundational principles established by the hospital's founder, Dr. Ernesto Contreras Sr.

Founding Principles

Our mission is based on two fundamental principles:

1. Do injury to no one.

2. Love your neighbor as yourself.

The first of these is fundamental to all medicine; the second is fundamental to our faith in the God who created the universe. Beyond that, these principles may seem simple, but they have a profound impact.

Why? Because Oasis of Hope physicians ask themselves three questions before they prescribe any medication or therapy:

1. Does the medical literature, my experience, and the counsel of my peers indicate that this medication has a high probability of helping the patient?

2. Will this medication I wish to prescribe harm the patient or cause side effects that outweigh any possible benefits?

3. If I had the same condition, would I take the same medication?

If you would like more information about cancer treatment at Oasis of Hope, please call us toll free or visit our Internet site, using the contact information below:

Oasis of Hope
1-888-500-HOPE
www.oasisofhope.com

NOTES

Introduction

1. National Cancer Institute, "National Cancer Act of 1971," http://www.dtp.nci.nih.gov/timeline/noflash/milestones/M4_Nixon.htm (accessed October 19, 2010).

2. American Cancer Society, "Cancer Facts and Figures 2010," http://www.cancer.org/research/cancerfactsfigures/cancerfactsfigures/cancer-facts-and-figures-2010 (accessed October 19, 2010).

Section 1
Preparing for Battle

1. See the Appendix, "The Oasis of Hope Cancer Treatment Centers."

Chapter 2
Genetic Instability

1. National Institutes of Health, "A Short History of the National Institutes of Health," Office of NIH History, http://history.nih.gov/exhibits/history/index.html (accessed October 20, 2010).

2. National Cancer Institute, "The 1971 National Cancer Act," http://rex.nci.nih.gov/massmedia/CANCER_RESRCH_WEBSITE/1971.html (accessed October 20, 2010).

3. Researchers believe that genetic instability is an integral component of human neoplasia1-3. Solid tumors undergo a variety of genetic alterations in their progression from normal to malignant cells. These changes happen through a series of multiple and abnormal genetic pathways. During cell replication, where precise DNA nucleotide (building block) pairing is essential, the normal genetic pathway can often be altered through translocations or gross chromosomal rearrangements (GCRs), asymmetric fragments, and large deletions, causing dangerous mismatches (mutations). Remember, DNA is a long chain of information. Genetic instability causes the long chains of information to be reproduced with errors; you might call them "genetic typos."

4. These two proteins, in order, are called hMSH2 and hMLH1.

5. Josef Rüschoff et al., "Aspirin Suppresses the Mutator Phenotype Associated With Hereditary Nonpolyposis Colorectal Cancer by Genetic Selection," *Proceedings of the National Academy of Sciences* 95 (September 15, 1998): 11301–11306.

6. Ibid.

7. This is according to Dr. Wu of the University of Texas M. D. Anderson Cancer Center, Houston (*Journal of the National Cancer Institute* 95, no. 7 (April 7, 2003): 540–547). Dr. B. N. Ames of UC–Berkeley has demonstrated that micronutrient deficiencies of vitamins B_{12}, B_6, C, E, folate, or niacin, and the minerals iron or zinc are a major cause of DNA damage. In fact, the genetic instability thus caused mimics that of gamma radiation (*Annals of the New York Academy of Sciences*, 1999). More than 20 percent of the population of the US intakes less than 50 percent of the recommended daily allowance (RDA) for each of these eight micronutrients. Dr. Wu says that low intake of folate has already been associated with a number of malignancies, including lung, cervical, colorectal, esophageal, brain, pancreatic, and breast cancers.

Chapter 3
The Immortal Cell

1. *Medical Post*, "The Immortal HeLa Cell Line" [named after first patient Henrietta Lacks], February 2, 1999.

2. N. W. Kim, M. A. Piatyszek, and K. R. Prowse, "Specific Association of Human Telomerase Activity with Immortal Cells and Cancer," *Science* 266, no. 5193 (1994): 2011–2015.

3. Jerry Shay, "Telomerase," http://claim.springer.de/EncRef/CancerResearch/samples/0001.htm. See also: L. R. Li et al., "Clinical Significance of Human Telomerase Reverse Transcriptase in Patients With Colon Cancer," *Ai Zheng* 23, Suppl. 1 (2004): 1502–1507. G. P. He et al., "Quantitative Detection of Telomerase Activity and Its Association With Clinicopathlogical Characteristics in Breast Cancer," *Ai Zheng* 23, no. 9 (2004): 1041–1046.

4. S. Hohaus et al., "Telomerase Activity in Human Laryngeal Squamous Cell Carcinomas," *Clinical Cancer Research* 2, no. 11 (1996): 1895–1900. E. Lusis and D. H. Gutmann, "Meningioma: An Update," *Curr Opin Neurol* 17(6) (2004): 687–692.

5. *PSA Rising Magazine*, "Vaccine Using Telomerase Tests on Prostate Cancer, Other Cancers, in San Diego and Paris," http://www.psa-rising.com/medicalpike/vaccine-telomerase-ucsd-april2000.htm. See also: B. Minev et al., "Cytotoxic T Cell Immunity Against Telomerase Reverse Transcriptase in Humans," *Proceedings of the National Academy of Science* 97, no. 9 (2000): 4796–4801. R. H. Vonderheiude et al., "Vaccination of Cancer Patients Against Telomerase Induces Functional Antitumor CD8+T Lymphocytes," *Clinical Cancer Research* 10, no. 3 (2004): 828–839.

6. Geron Pharmaceuticals, "Presentations on Geron's Telomerase Inhibitor at AACR Special Conference," March 2, 2010, http://www.geron.com/media/pressview.aspx?id=1213 (accessed October 21, 2010).

7. Fred Hutchinson Cancer Research Center, http://www.fhcrc.org. See also: Ivy Greenwell, "Green Tea," *LE Magazine*, http://www.lef.org/magazine/mag99/june99-report2.html (accessed October 21, 2010).

Chapter 4
How Cancer Fights

1. J. Liu et al., "DNA Methylation Affects Cell Proliferation, Cortisol Secretion and Steroidogenic Gene Expression in Human Adrenocortical NCI-H295R Cells," *Journal of Molecular Endocrinology* 33, no. 3 (2004): 651–662. B. Malfoy, "The Revival of DNA Methylation," *Jounal of Cell Science* 113, pt 22 (2000): 3887–3888.

2. There is also evidence that appropriate chromosome structure may be affected by methylation and that human diseases, including cancer, are affected by changes in chromatin structure.

3. Aberrant DNA methylation is now recognized as a contributing factor in a number of human diseases. Since the late 1980s, numerous studies have described abnormal methylation of DNA in tumors and transformed cells. It is well known that carcinogens such as dichlorodiphenyltrichloroethane (DDT), phenobarbital, arsenic, zinc deficiency, and cigarette smoke alter methyl metabolism and/or DNA methylation. Understanding the mechanism of methylation might also help explain the increased risk of cancer in smokers. For example, squamous cell carcinoma of the lung is characterized by increased abnormal DNA methylation. Aberrant methylation may occur near or within a tumor-suppressor gene that silences its anticancer activity, obviously increasing the risk of developing malignant tumors.

4. Brown's research may have uncovered at least one of the ways resistance occurs and a potentially effective way of reversing the process. This research group has discovered that cancer cells turn chemotherapy resistant because several key genes that allow cancer cells to be responsive to chemo are summarily switched off by "bad" DNA methylation. Decitabine switches the genes back on, making cancer cells once again sensitive to the effects of the chemotherapy.

5. K. Appleton et al., "Phase I and Pharmacodynamic Trial of the DNA Methyltransferase Inhibitor Decitabine and Carboplatin in Solid Tumors," *Journal of Clinical Oncology*, 25, no. 29 (October 10, 2007): 4603–4609.

6. Indeed, epidemiologic studies have established that a low intake of vegetables rich in folate is associated with increased risk for colon cancer. Conversely, a high intake of folate derived from either food or from supplements is associated with decreased risk for colon cancer and adenoma, which is a precursor for colon cancer.

This information is not new. Salmon and Copeland showed that methyl-deficient diets caused liver cancer in rats as long ago as 1946. And in 1954, Wilgram et al. showed that choline deficiency caused atherosclerosis and death in young rats. The importance of methyl groups in avoiding liver cancer was later more clearly shown and extended by Dr. Lionel Poirier and coworkers.

Also, dietary deficiencies of folate, methionine, vitamin B_{12}, and choline have been associated with genetic abnormalities, chemical toxicity on aberrant DNA methylation, and increased cancer risk. It is also known that folate and vitamin B_{12} are involved in the generation of methyl groups for DNA methylation, and that nutritional deficiencies, with respect to these vitamins, may encourage aberrant DNA methylation. More so, interactions of folate with other dietary factors that influence methylation, such as alcohol, vitamin B_{12}, and methionine, also appear to influence cancer risk. For example, low folate intake and high alcohol intake increases the risk of adenomas (colon cancer precursors) as well as breast cancer.

Resistance, even for multiple chemo drugs, can be undermined with a diet rich in folate and other vitamins. We have been able to use low-dose chemotherapy with success against tumors deemed resistant when patients are given diets rich in methyl-donor foods. Not only do the patients experience tumor destruction, but they also suffer very few side effects.

One additional note for the techno-savvy. A public database for DNA methylation has now been established. At the time this book was written, the database contained methylation patterns, profiles, and total methylation content data for 41 species, 117 tissues, and 56 phenotypes, from a total of 1,432 experiments. More than half of the data for human tissues refers to DNA methylation in cancer cells. MethDB has an open structure and can be extended and adapted easily. It is also linked to other databases on the Web, including PubMed, GenBank at http://genome.imb-jena.de/methtools/. It is also worth noting that fairly small changes in nutrient levels caused dramatic developmental changes in mice, according to *Molecular and Cellular Biology* for August 1, 2003.

Chapter 5
Three Major Weapons of Conventional Medicine

1. American Cancer Society, "Major Issues to Be Discussed at the February Market Forces Meeting," November 11, 1998, viewed at http://www.charitywire.com/charity6/02321.html (accessed October 21, 2010).

2. American Cancer Society, "Cancer Facts and Figures 2009," http://www.cancer.org/acs/groups/content/@nho/documents/document/500809webpdf.pdf (accessed October 21, 2010).

3. International Agency for Research on Cancer, "World Cancer Report," December 10, 2008, http://www.iarc.fr/en/publications/pdfs-online/wcr/index.php (accessed October 21, 2010).

4. ScienceDaily.com, "Cancer Projected to Become Leading Cause of death Worldwide in 2010," December 9, 2008, http://www.sciencedaily.com/releases/2008/12/081209111516.htm (accessed October 21, 2010).

5. See the appendix, "The Oasis of Hope Cancer Treatment Centers."

6. Ralph W. Moss, "Chemo's Berlin Wall Crumbles," *Cancer Chronicles* 7 (December 1990): http://www.ralphmoss.com/html/ChemoBerlin.shtml (accessed October 21, 2010).

7. Ibid.

8. H. H. Hansen, "Advanced Non-Small-Cell Lung Cancer: To Treat or Not to Treat," *Journal of Clinical Oncology* (November 1, 1987): 1711–1712.

9. J. C. Bailar III and Elaine M. Smith, "Progress Against Cancer?" *New England Journal of Medicine* 314, no. 19 (1986): 1226–1232.

10. Moss, "Chemo's Berlin Wall Crumbles."

11. Bailar and Smith, "Progress Against Cancer?"

12. J. C. Bailar III, "Cancer Undefeated," *New England Journal of Medicine* 336, no. 22 (May 29, 1997): 1569–1574.

13. M. V. Peter, "Wedge Resection With or Without Radiation in Early Breast Cancer," *International Journal of Radiation Oncology and Biological Physicology* 2, no. 11/12 (November/December 1977): 1151–1156.

Chapter 6
Consider These Alternative Therapies

1. IMOS Italia, "Ossigeno Ozono Terapia," http://www.imos-italia.it/index .php?middle=ozono (accessed December 20, 2004).

2. Autohemotherapy is the process of bringing small quantities of blood into contact with ozone. Ozone therapy is performed each year on several hundred thousand patients around the world, mostly in Russia, Poland, Greece, Germany, Switzerland, Italy, Austria, Belgium, and Cuba. The medical ozone used in this therapy is an O_2/O_3 mixture with a low ozone concentration. The ozone generators used to produce this mixture are incredibly precise.

Autohemotherapy is typically performed in one of two ways. The standard technique is to withdraw 150–250 ml of blood and expose it to a O_2/O_3 mixture at a specified ozone concentration, followed by intravenous reinfusion of this blood into the patient. At the Oasis of Hope, we have the option of running an extracorporeal loop to ozonate all of the patient's blood. This second technique involves automatically running the blood through a continuous recirculating device, which mixes ozone and blood in a closed loop before reinfusing it.

The results from two very recent studies proved the safety and effectiveness of the ozonation of blood in humans. No significant changes in blood chemistry or other parameters were found. The patients felt no particular sensations during treatment. The treatment session was followed by a feeling of well-being and euphoria lasting several hours. Most important, there was a total lack of side effects. The authors conclude that blood ozonation is clinically valid, without side effects, and that this treatment could be useful when orthodox therapies have failed in at least four areas: infectious diseases, vascular disorders, degenerative diseases (particularly metastatic cancer), and pathologies related to immune depression.

3. A. Raa et al., "Hyperoxia Retards Growth and Induces Apoptosis and Loss of Glands and Blood Vessels in DMBA-Induced Rat Mammary Tumors," *BMC Cancer* 7 (January 30, 2007): 23.

4. Named for Dr. E. K. Knott, who refined the original therapy.

5. G. Grick and A. Linke, "Ultraviolet Irradiation of the Blood; Its Development and Current Status," *Z Arztl Fortbild* 80, no. 11 (1986): 441–444.

6. A. V. Marochkov, V. A. Doronin, and N. N. Kravtsov, "Complications in Ultraviolet Irradiation of the Blood," *Anesteziologiia I Reanimatologiia* 4 (1990): 55–56.

7. There is a recent modification to standard ECP therapy, called *trans-immunization therapy* (TI). This is a way of tailoring the therapy to individual patients. The first major difference is that the white blood cells are cultured overnight after exposure to the 8-MOP and ultraviolet light. The white blood cells called monocytes transform immature dendritic cells. These immature dendritic cells are aggressive and can internalize apoptotic cancer cells. So, the white blood cells are cultured overnight with a solution of dead cancer cells, removed from the patient in surgery. The immature dendritic cells ingest these cancer cells, stimulating a "specific" antitumor immunity. When the antigen-loaded dendritic cells mature, they are intravenously returned to the patient and stimulate a "personalized antitumor vaccine."

8. With respect to cancer, dendritic cells initiate an antitumor response from the immune system by identifying malignant cells as a target. Treatment with ECP therapy also increases the production of the cytokines the immune system uses to kill malignant cells. Specifically, the therapy increases production of interferon and interleukin-2.

Without question, the most important anticancer cytokine is interleukin-2. A cancer immunotherapy requires the transfer of tumor-distinctive antigens from malignant cells to "professional" antigen-presenting cells, like dendritic cells, to initiate clinically relevant antitumor responses from the immune system, like the production of interleukin.

9. L. A. Sauer, R. T. Dauchy, and D. E. Blask, "Polyunsaturated Fatty Acids, Melatonin, and Cancer," *Biochemical Pharmacolology* 61, no. 12 (2001): 1455–1462.

10. P. Lissoni, "Is There a Role for Melatonin in Supportive Care?" *Support Care Cancer* 10, no. 2 (2002): 110–116.

11. Ibid.

12. Ibid.

13. Ibid.

14. P. Lissoni et al., "Neuroimmunomodulation in Medical Oncology: Application of Psychoneuroimmunology With Subcutaneous Low-Dose IL-2 and

the Pineal Hormone Melatonin in Patients With Untreatable Metastatic Solid Tumors," *Anticancer Research* 2B (March/April 2008): 1377–1381.

15. M. Kondo and M. F. McCarty, "Rationale for a Novel Immunotherapy of Cancer With Allogeneic Lymphocyte Infusion," *Medical Hypotheses* 3 (November 15, 1984): 241–277.

16. H. J. Symons et al., "The Allogeneic Effect Revisited: Exogenous Help for Endogenous, Tumor-Specific T Cells," *Biology Blood Marrow Transplant* 14, no. 5 (May 2008): 499–509.

Chapter 8
Avoid Toxic Foods and Harmful Substances

1. Information obtained from the Internet by searching the *Guinness Book of World Records* with Texis, Thunderstone Document Retrieval and Management. Also found at http://www.cerias.purdue.edu/homes/spaf/Yucks/V3/msg00030 .html (accessed October 22, 2010).

2. Joseph D. Beasley, *The Betrayal of Health: The Impact of Nutrition, Environment and Lifestyle on Illness in America* (New York: Random House, 1991), 85.

3. Ibid., 108.

4. Robert M. Kradjian, "Milk, the Natural Thing?" *Newlife* (November–December 1994).

5. Ibid.

6. Ibid.

7. Francisco Contreras, et al., *Health in the 21st Century: Will Doctors Survive?* (Chula Vista, CA: Interpacific Press, 1997), 107.

8. Ibid., 108.

9. Marguerite Holloway, "Dioxin Indictment," *Scientific American* 270 (January 1994): 25.

10. Theo Colburn, *Our Stolen Future* (New York: Penguin Group, 1997), 150–152.

11. Richard M. Sharpe and Niels S. Skakkebaek, "Are Estrogens Involved in Falling Sperm Counts and Disorders of the Male Reproductive Tract?" *Lancet* 341 (May 29, 1993): 1392–1395.

12. L. A. Brinton, "Ways That Women May Reduce Their Possible Risk of Breast Cancer," *Journal of the National Cancer Institute* (1994).

13. Ralph W. Moss, "Cancer Risks Lurk in Hot Dogs and Burgers," *Cancer Chronicles* (July 1994).

14. Susan Preston-Martin et al., "Maternal Consumption of Cured Meats and Vitamins in Relation to Pediatric Brain Tumors," *Cancer Epidemiology, Biomarkers and Prevention* 5, no. 8 (August 1996): 599–605.

15. Beasley, *The Betrayal of Health*, 106.

16. Julian Whitaker, *Health and Healing* 7 (November 1977); also, "The Truth About Olestra," Army Physical Fitness Research Institute, U.S. Army War College, http://WWW.carlisle.army.mil/apfri/the_truth_about_olestra.htm (accessed December 20, 2004).

17. Beasley, *The Betrayal of Health*, 106.

18. Kian Liu et al., "Dietary Cholesterol, Fat, and Fiber, and Cancer Colon Mortality: An Analysis of International Data," *Lancet* 2 (October 13, 1979): 782–785. E. L. Wynder, "Dietary Habits and Cancer Epidemiology," *Cancer* 43, 5 Suppl (May 1979): 1955–1961.

19. T. D. Wilkins and A. S. Hackman, "Two Patterns of Neutral Steroid Conversion in the Feces of Normal North Americans," *Cancer Research* 34 (1974): 2250–2254.

20. Stephen Shoenthaler, "Institutional Nutritional Policies and Criminal Behavior," *Nutrition Today* 20, no. 3 (1985): 16.

21. Stephen Shoenthaler, "Diet and Crime: An Empirical Examination of the Value of Nutrition in the Control and Treatment of Incarcerated Juvenile Offenders," *International Journal of Biosocial Research* 4, no. 1 (1983): 25–39.

22. Beasley, *The Betrayal of Health*, 76.

23. Ibid., 77.

24. The China Project was a research project examining the relationship of diet to health by studying the way diet and life patterns affect health. It was based in rural China and is considered the most comprehensive database on the multiple causes of disease ever compiled.

25. T. Colin Campbell and Christine Cox, *The China Project: Inside Our Living Laboratory* (n.p.: New Century Nutrition, 1996), 23.

Chapter 9
Eat Foods That Can Heal You

1. A. P. Simopoulos, "The Mediterranean Diets: What Is So Special About the Diet of Greece? The Scientific Evidence," *Journal of Nutrition* 131, 11 Suppl (November 2001): 3065S–3073S.

2. H. Nakagawa, "Resveratrol Inhibits Human Breast Cancer Cell Growth and May Mitigate the Effect of Linoleic Acid, a Potent Breast Cancer Cell Stimulator," *Journal of Cancer Research and Clinical Oncology* 127, no. 4 (April 2001): 258–264.

3. B. D. Gehm, "Resveratrol, a Polyphenolic Compound Found in Grapes and Wine, Is an Agonist for the Estrogen Receptor," *Proceedings of the National Academy of Sciences of the United States* 94, no. 25 (December 9, 1997): 14138–14143.

4. D. J. Jenkins et al., "Effect of Almonds on Insulin Secretion and Insulin Resistance in Nondiabetic Hyperlipidemic Subjects: A Randomized Controlled Crossover Trial," *Metabolism* 57, no. 7 (July 2008): 882–887.

5. E. Giovannucci, "A Prospective Study of Tomato Products, Lycopene, and Prostate Cancer Risk," *Journal of the National Cancer Institute* 94, no. 5 (March 6, 2002): 391–398.

6. M. Jang, "Cancer Chemopreventive Activity of Resveratrol," *Drugs Uner Experimental and Clinical Research* 25, no. 2–3 (1999): 65–77.

7. Remember, cancer occurs when there is an undesirable change in the nucleus of the cells in the body—specifically in the DNA, resulting in an accelerating process of uncontrollable, inappropriate cell growth in the body. The cancerous cell is the most toxic type that can be in the living body. It is believed that we all have them; therefore, we must do whatever is necessary to keep them in remission before they can become active cancers. But if they are already active cancers, our job is to provide the optimal conditions, through dietary and lifestyle changes, to allow the body to heal itself. Is that really possible? My good friends at Hallelujah Acres have received hundreds of testimonies from all over the world from people who have seen their body's warning signs of disease disappear after following the Hallelujah diet and lifestyle recommendations for a reasonable length of time.

8. Epidemiologic and animal studies have associated certain food plants with pronounced reductions in cancer risk. Among such plants are cruciferous (mustard family) vegetables such as broccoli, cabbage, cauliflower, and brussels sprouts. What characteristics of these vegetables might protect against carcinogenesis? Brassica vegetables contain little fat, are low in energy, and are good sources of vitamins, minerals, and fiber—all linked to cancer protection. They also contain a large number of phytochemicals, some of which protect against carcinogenesis in various in vitro and animal testing systems. Recent research results also show that consumption of cruciferous vegetables, particularly broccoli, plays an important role in decreasing the risk of breast cancer in premenopausal women.

9. Joel Fuhrman, *Eat to Live: The Revolutionary Formula for Fast and Sustained Weight Loss* (New York: Little, Brown and Company, 2003), 59.

10. S. Agarwal and A. V. Rao, "Tomato Lycopene and Its Role in Human Health and Chronic Disease," *Canadian Medical Association Journal* 163, no. 6 (2000): 739–744. S. Franceshi et al., "Tomatoes and the Risk of Digestive-Tract Cancers," *International Journal of Cancer* 59 (1994): 181–184.

11. E. Giovannucci, "Tomato-Based Products, Lycopene, and Cancer: Review of the Epidemiologic Literature," *Journal of the National Cancer Institute* 91 (1999): 317–331.

12. Q-Y Lu et al., "Inverse Associations Between Plasma Lycopene and Other Carotenoids and Prostate Cancer," *Cancer Epidemiology, Biomarkers and Prevention* 10, no. 7 (July 2001): 749–756.

13. N. T. Thuy, P. He, and H. Takeuchi, "Comparative Effect of Dietary Olive, Safflower, and Linseed Oils on Spontaneous Liver Tumorigenesis in

C3H/He Mice," *Journal of Nutritional Science and Vitaminology* 47, no. 5 (2001): 363–366.

14. H. E. Kirschner, *Live Food Juices* (n.p.: Cancer Book House, 1980), 20–21.

15. Data from P. M. Kris-Etherton et al., "Polyunsaturated Fatty Acids in the Food Chain in the United States," *American Journal of Clinical Nutrition* 71, Suppl (2000): 179S-188S.

Chapter 10
Take Advantage of Nature's Pharmacy

1. G. Li et al., "Antiproliferative Effects of Garlic Constituents on Cultured Human Breast Cancer Cells," *Oncology Reports* 2 (1995): 787–791.

2. C. Borek, "Antioxidant Health Effects of Aged Garlic Extract," *Journal of Nutrition* 131, no. 3s (March 2001):1010S–1015S.

3. K. Folkers et al., "Survival of Cancer Patients on Therapy With Coenzyme Q$_{10}$," *Biochemical and Biophysical Research Communications* 192, no. 1 (April 15, 1993): 241–245.

4. K. Lockwood et al., "Progress on Therapy of Breast Cancer With Coenzyme Q$_{10}$ and the Regression of Metastases," *Biochemical and Biophysical Research Communications* 212, no. 1 (July 6, 1995): 172–177.

5. The first article saying that silymarin was evaluated as a chemopreventive agent comes from 1991: R. G. Mehta and R. C. Moon, "Characterization of Effective Chemopreventive Agents in Mammary Gland in Vitro Using an Initiation-Promotion Protocol," *Anticancer Research* 11, no. 2 (1991): 593–596.

6. S. K. Katiyar, "Silymarin and Skin Cancer Prevention: Anti-Inflammatory, Antioxidant and Immunomodulatory Effects," *International Journal of Oncology* 26, no. 1 (2005): 169–176.

7. M. Kaur et al., "Silibinin Suppresses Growth and Induces Apoptotic Death of Human Colorectal Carcinoma LoVo Cells in Culture and Tumor Xenograft," *Molecular Cancer Therapy* 8, no. 8 (August 2009): 2366–2374. R. P. Singh et al., "Silibinin Suppresses Growth of Human Prostate Carcinoma PC-3 Orthotopic Xenograft via Activation of Extracellular Signal-Regulated Kinase 1/2 and Inhibition of Signal Transducers and Activators of Transcription Signaling," *Clinical Cancer Research* 15, no. 2 (January 15, 2009): 613–621.

8. W. Cui, F. Gu, and H. Q. Hu, "Effects and Mechanisms of Silibinin on Human Hepatocellular Carcinoma Xenografts in Nude Mice," *World Journal of Gastroenterology* 15, no. 1) (April 28, 2009): 1943–1950.

9. G. Deep et al., "Isosilibinin Inhibits Advanced Human Prostate Cancer Growth in Athymic Nude Mice: Comparison With Silymarin and Silibinin," *International Journal of Cancer* 123, no. 12 (December 15, 2008): 2750–2758. K. Raina et al., "Stage-Specific Inhibitory Effects and Associated Mechanisms of Silibinin on Tumor Progression and Metastasis in Transgenic Adenocarcinoma

of the Mouse Prostate Model," *Cancer Research* 68, no. 16 (August 15, 2008): 6822–6830. R. P. Singh et al., "Oral Silibinin Inhibits in Vivo Human Bladder Tumor Xenograft Growth Involving Down-Regulation of Survivin," *Clinical Cancer Research* 14, no. 1 (January 1, 2008): 300–308. R. P. Singh et al., "Suppression of Advanced Human Prostate Tumor Growth in Athymic Mice by Silibinin Feeding Is Associated With Reduced Cell Proliferation, Increased Apoptosis, and Inhibition of Angiogenesis," *Cancer Epidemiology, Biomarkers and Prevention* 12, no. 9 (September 2003): 933–939. R. P. Singh et al., "Dietary Feeding of Silibinin Inhibits Advance Human Prostate Carcinoma Growth in Athymic Nude Mice and Increases Plasma Insulin-Like Growth Factor-Binding Protein-3 Levels," *Cancer Research* 62, no. 11 (June 1, 2002): 3063–3069.

10. Singh et al., "Oral Silibinin Inhibits in Vivo Human Bladder Tumor Xenograft Growth Involving Down-Regulation of Survivin."

11. R. P. Singh et al., "Oral Silibinin Inhibits Lung Tumor Growth in Athymic Nude Mice and Forms a Novel Chemocombination with Doxorubicin Targeting Nuclear Factor KappaB-Mediated Inducible Chemoresistance," *Clinical Cancer Research* 10, no. 24 (December 15, 2004): 8641–8647.

12. Proteolytic enzymes act as immunomodulators by raising the impaired immunocytotoxicity of leukocytes against tumor cells from patients and by inducing the production of distinct cytokines such as tumor necrosis factor, interleukin (IL)-1, IL-6, and IL-8. Not all of these antitumoral activities depend on the proteolytic activity of enzymes, but on their effects on the modulation of immune functions, including the anti-inflammatory activities and their potential to accelerate wound healing. Proteolytic enzymes are also used in the treatment of pancreatic insufficiency, cystic fibrosis, digestive problems, viral infections, surgical traumas, autoimmune disorders, and sports injuries. Ultimately, enzyme therapy can significantly clear "immune complexes" (combinations of antibodies and antigens) from the body. When the body is incapable of releasing these immune complexes, an inflammatory process begins that can lead to serious disease, often of the autoimmune type. Dramatic results have been reported with the use of enzyme therapy in such diseases as rheumatoid arthritis, multiple sclerosis, and systemic lupus erythematosus.

Chapter 11
Understand the Brain-Body Cancer Connection

1. The discovery of this class of biochemicals has an unusual and interesting history. In the 1960s, biomedical researchers studying the causes and effects of opium addiction detected what they suspected were opiate receptors in brain tissue. Since it seemed quite unlikely that humans would contain a specific receptor designed for a chemical derived from the poppy plant, the researchers focused their attention on biochemicals that might be synthesized in the brain itself.

In the early 1970s, several small peptides were isolated. These appeared to possess natural analgesic properties, and they were collectively termed *enkephalins* and *endorphins*.

The modification of neural transmissions by these biochemicals now appears to be responsible for the insensitivity to pain experienced by individuals under conditions of great stress or shock. The effectiveness of analgesic opiate derivatives, such as opium, morphine, and heroin, is an accidental side effect that derives from the ability of these substances to bind to neurohormone receptors, despite their very different structures.

The pituitary gland synthesizes hormone precursors or prohormones. This peptide is cleaved in the pituitary to generate ACTH and beta-lipotropin, while other processes in the central nervous system produce endorphins and enkephalins, along with some other products. Endorphins are most heavily released in the human body during stressful events or in moments of great pain. However, the amount of endorphins released by individuals varies, such that an occurrence that stimulates significant neurohormone secretion in some people will not necessarily do so in others.

William Glasser, MD, a prominent psychiatrist and educator, wrote a book in 1976 entitled *Positive Addiction* in which he describes the body's reaction to physical pain from the trauma that frequent running causes to an athlete's joints. Pain prompts their brain to release endorphins and adrenaline into their blood to anesthetize them to this pain and enhance performance. Endorphine, a natural painkiller, acts like a narcotic, not only to dull the pain but also to cause what is now called a "runner's high."

2. Programs, policies, and procedures of the William Glasser Institute, California.

3. W. Glasser, "Choice Therapy," http://www.wglasser.com/index.php?option =com_content&task=view&id=12&Itemid=27 (accessed October 22, 2010).

4. Gerald Tortura and Sandra Grabowski, *Principles of Anatomy and Physiology*, 8th edition (New York: Wiley and Sons, n.d.).

5. Quoted by Bart P. Billings, "Feeling the Music Can Be Dangerous to Your Health: A Comprehensive Review," http://www.omnisonic.com/bbillings.html.

6. Janice R. Kiecolt-Glaser and Ronald Glaser, two leading researchers in this field, summarized the research in *Psychoneuroimmunology*. They cite many studies that report, with remarkable consistency across populations and different kinds of events, that stressful life events called "major negative life changes," such as bereavement, divorce, depression, chronic stress, and academic stress, all depress immune function and put people at greater risk for a variety of diseases. In particular, events associated with the loss of important personal relationships appear to put individuals at greater risk. The Glasers have found that bereaved people have higher mortality in general and a higher incidence of cancer in particular

than controls do, and that divorce has even greater health risks associated with it than bereavement.

7. Doctors in general, and oncologists in particular, reject any participation in providing any hope above what statistics offer. Any other hope is labeled as false. I have stated before that there is either hope or no hope, and that patients are always entitled to it.

8. Recent advances in psychoneuroendocrinological knowledge have shown that the perception of pleasure is mainly mediated by the dopaminergic pathways in the brain, which now can be measured by evaluating blood levels of cortisol and other hormones in response to stimulation with opiod chemicals such as apomorphine.

Italian researchers administered apomorphine to cancer patients and documented possible cancer-related neuroendocrine anomalies, which could explain the psychological status of the patients. These cancer patients showed no increase in the hormones expected to rise due to apomorphine stimulation, regardless of the type of tumor and how advanced it was.

The results of this study show that the neoplastic disease is characterized by neurochemical alterations involving pleasure-related dopaminergic pathways, which are more evident in the metastatic disease, without particular differences in relation to tumor type.

Therefore, the psychological condition of cancer patients would not depend only on psychological factors, but also it could be due at least in part to cancer-related neuroendocrine alterations.

But the more we study these facts, the more scientists are convinced that there is no "cancer personality." A psychological profile does not doom people to develop cancer. At the Oasis of Hope Hospital we have experienced tremendous turnaround of patients who felt hopeless but changed their attitudes and had tumor regression as a side effect.

9. Campbell et al., *Scientists Say Vitamin C May Alleviate the Body's Response to Stress*, American Chemical Society, August 23, 1999.

Chapter 12
Cope With Stress

1. J. Casseday, B. McClelland, and C. Yaros, "Teen Suicide: Parents Echo Cry for Help," *Tampa Tribune*, February 29, 2004.

2. Roger Bannister, *The Four-Minute Mile*, 50th anniversary edition (Guilford, CT: Lyons Press, 1955, 1981, 2004), 171.

3. From the foreword by Patch Adams in Francisco Contreras, *The Hope of Living Cancer Free* (Lake Mary, FL: Siloam, 1999), xi.

Chapter 13
Think Positive Thoughts

1. TheDenverChannel.com, "Study: Depression, Sadness Weaken Immune System," September 2, 2003, http://www.thedenverchannel.com/print/2448536/detail.html (accessed October 22, 2010).

Chapter 14
Surround Yourself With Positive Friends

1. P. A. Henderson, "Psychosocial Adjustment of Adult Cancer Survivors: Their Needs and Counselor Interventions," *Journal of Counseling and Development* 1, no. 3 (January/February 1997): 189.

2. N. M. Lindberg and D. K. Wellisch, "Identification of Traumatic Stress Reactions in Women at Increased Risk for Breast Cancer," *Psychosomatics* 45, no. 1 (January/February 2004): 7.

3. M. Lloyd-Williams, "Depression—the Hidden Symptom in Advanced Cancer," *Journal of the Royal Society of Medicine* 96, no. 12 (December 1993): 577.

4. C. G. Shields and S. J. Rousseau, "A Pilot Study of an Intervention for Breast Cancer Survivors and Their Spouses," *Family Process* 43, no. 1 (2004): 95–107.

Chapter 15
Soul-Searching Time: Find the Will to Live

1. Bernie S. Siegel, *Love, Medicine and Miracles* (New York: Harper and Row Publishing, 1986).

Chapter 16
Laugh All the Way to the Bank

1. Billings, "Feeling the Music Can Be Dangerous to Your Health: A Comprehensive Review."

Chapter 18
Tap Into the Power of Hope

1. H. G. Koenig et al., "Religiosity and Remission Depression in Medically Ill Patients," *American Journal of Psychiatry* 155 (April 1998): 536–542.

2. R. C. Byrd, "Positive Therapeutic Effects of Intercessory Prayer in a Coronary Care Unit Population," *Southern Medical Journal* 81, no. 7 (1998): 826–829.

Chapter 19
Don't Overlook Prayer Therapy

1. Byrd, "Positive Therapeutic Effects of Intercessory Prayer in a Coronary Care Unit Population."

2. Duke Medicine News and Communications, "Prayer, Noetic Studies Feasible; Results Indicate Benefit," DukeHealth.org, Nov. 3, 2004, www.dukehealth.org/health_library/news/5056 (accessed November 1, 2010).

3. E. Braunwald, "Coronary-Artery Surgery at the Crossroads," *New England Journal of Medicine* 297, no. 12 (September 22, 1977): 661–663.

Chapter 20
Access Your Heavenly Resources

1. Contreras, *Health in the 21st Century.*

2. Leo Buscaglia, *Living, Loving and Learning* (New York: Ballantine Books, 1985).

3. Siegel, *Love, Medicine and Miracles*, 182–183.

4. Ibid., 244.

ABOUT THE AUTHORS

Francisco Contreras, MD

Francisco Contreras, MD, has gained worldwide attention in part for his skill and experience as a cancer surgeon but also for his ability to integrate natural therapies with orthodox medicine in pursuit of total well-being for his patients.

Dr. Contreras received his premed training at Pasadena College, Pasadena, California. He went on to complete medical school at the Universidad Autónoma de Mexico in 1978. After a year of social medical service, he traveled with his bride, Rosa Alicia Contreras, to Vienna to specialize in surgical oncology at one of the world's finest medical schools, the Chirurgische Universitatsklinik, recognized for producing such renowned doctors as Dr. Sigmund Freud. After completing his specialty, Dr. Contreras returned to Mexico to begin work with his father at the Oasis of Hope Hospital in 1983.

Patients have come to the Oasis of Hope from more than fifty-five countries. Now Dr. Contreras is taking the combined experience of forty-eight years of medical practice and more than one hundred thousand patients to the world. He shares his vision of hope through television, radio, and conferences, including the World Congress on Breast Cancer. He has met with top officials, including the chairman of the Japanese FDA and the Georgia State House of Representatives.

Dr. Contreras believes that most people fall prey to disease for lack of knowledge. He believes that education can have a greater impact in improving the health of humanity than research breakthroughs. This conviction compels him to travel extensively to share his knowledge with others. As a part of his mission, he has written twelve books on cancer, joint health, menopause, antiaging, the secret healing power contained within tomatoes and grapes, heart health, and the modern-day adversaries of health.

Dr. Contreras also founded the Francisco Contreras Clinical Research Organization, which has conducted a number of clinical trials, has formulated unique natural food supplements, and has designed protocols for clinical trials on new drugs. One of the newest pharmaceuticals that has been registered in Mexico by Dr. Contreras's team is PERFTEC, the only registered blood substitute in the world.

Daniel E. Kennedy, MC, MBA, BA

Daniel E. Kennedy is the chief executive officer of the Oasis of Hope Health Group. He has been counseling cancer patients since 1993. His background in business and counseling has enabled him to advance the Oasis of Hope Hospital treatment approach based on the total needs of a patient's body, mind, and spirit.

Mr. Kennedy holds a Master of Counseling, an MBA, and a BA in liberal arts. He is a member of the Association of Oncology Social Work and is certified as a Christian marriage and family therapist by the American Society of Christian Therapists.

In 1998, Mr. Kennedy founded the Worldwide Cancer Prayer Day to urge people to unite in prayer and turn to God for healing (www.cancerprayernetwork.com). He was inspired to start this prayer day after his father was diagnosed with cancer, and healed, in 1997. His father continues to be well.

Mr. Kennedy has written four books on healing and cancer and has been published in various Christian magazines and newspapers. He speaks in conferences in the United States and Europe and is a frequent guest on television and radio programs. His topics include "Emotional and Spiritual Victory Over Cancer," "Finding God's Hand in a Cancer Crisis," "Overcoming an Identity Crisis," and "Prayer Therapy." He is also a music minister and has had one album distributed by the number one label in Latin America, "CanZion." He has ministered with music, counseling and preaching throughout the United States, Mexico, the United Kingdom, Europe, Africa, and Asia. To find out more about Daniel Kennedy ministries, please visit www.danielkennedy.info. You can also go to the iTunes app store and download the application "Daniel Kennedy" to your iPhone.

INDEX

A

Abel, Dr. Ulrich 34–35

active hexose correlated compound (AHCC) 59, 101

Adams, Patch 11, 116

adrenaline 28, 106–107

aged garlic extract 99–100

American Cancer Society (ACS) 32–33

arthritis 72, 77

asbestos 60

B

Bailar III, Dr. J. C. 34–35

B cells 58

bovine growth hormone 72

C

"Cancer Facts & Figures 2009" 32–33

Cancer Prayer Day 180–181, 214

carcinogens 59, 66, 70, 90, 100

chemotherapy 2, 5–6, 25–26, 29, 31, 33–35, 39–40, 59, 82, 101, 137, 170, 187

    and gene amplification 27

    and resistance to 53

    barrier 27

    deficiencies of 45

    detoxification 27

    efficacy of 2, 34

    mutations 27

    negative side effects of 40

    neutralization 27

    resistance to 26–27

    side effects of 48, 101, 104

China Project, the 81

cholesterol 47, 79, 102, 108–109, 111, 157, 185

    and hormone production 108

coenzyme Q_{10} (CoQ_{10}) 102

Cytomegalovirus (CMV) 61

D

depression 61, 67, 110, 114, 117, 137–138

diabetes 32, 72, 77, 161

digestive enzymes 104

    pancreatic enzymes 103–104

    proteolytic enzymes 104

DNA 7, 16, 18, 19–20, 191

    damage 20, 54

    damaging agents 19

    instability 54

    metabolism 29

    methylation 27–29

    mutation 57–58

    of cancer 16

    protection of 54

    repair 20, 27, 52, 90

E

endorphins 106, 111–112, 151–152, 170, 186

estrogen 67, 72–74, 79

    estrogen-like 72–73

    estrogenic chemicals 79

    estrogenic effect 72–73

F

Finsen, Dr. Niels Ryberg 49

folate (folic acid) 20, 29, 66, 69

Frankl, Viktor 143–144, 168

Fuhrman, Dr. Joel 90

G

genetic instability 15–16, 18–20, 25, 54

Gerson therapy, the 89

glucose 108

    glucose intolerance 72